Why Mums Don't Jump

Why Mums Don't Jump

Ending the Pelvic Floor Taboo

Helen Ledwick

Illustrations by Cat Pearson

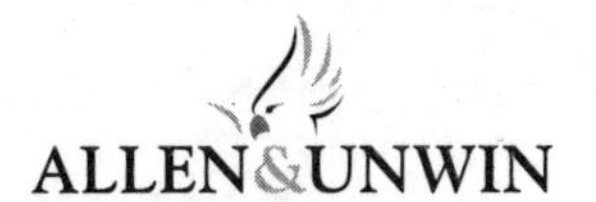

First published in Great Britain in trade paperback in 2023 by Allen & Unwin

Allen & Unwin
c/o Atlantic Books
Ormond House
26–27 Boswell Street
London WC1N 3JZ

Phone: 020 7269 1610
Email: UK@allenandunwin.com
Web: www.allenandunwin.com/uk

A CIP catalogue record for this book is available from the British Library.

Trade paperback ISBN 978 1 83895 849 7
E-book ISBN 978 1 83895 850 3

Printed in Great Britain by TJ Books Limited

10 9 8 7 6 5 4 3 2 1

For Dad,
who never gave up.

Contents

Introduction

'Mummy has a broken bottom,' my son tells anyone at seemingly every possible opportunity. 'My sister came out of her tummy. But I came out of her bottom and it broke.'

That's what happens when you try to explain to a preschooler why they should absolutely not peep around the curtain during a hospital appointment for a ruined pelvic floor. A gynaecological investigation needs no witnesses, thank you. If you sit there and watch CBeebies you can have all the sweets later.

He may not be exactly anatomically correct, but you have to admire his ability to share this news so freely. He isn't at all bothered by the taboo that surrounds leaks and lumps after childbirth – pelvic floor problems that stop us from trampolining and then sometimes change *absolutely everything* about the way we live our lives and feel about ourselves.

Incontinence. Prolapse. Pelvic pain. We don't like to even

speak these words because society has taught us that it's all too shameful or that it's just a part of motherhood to be endured. For most of us, it comes so far out of left field that we're reeling from the idea of it, let alone ready to bust it out over dinner. I get it. I went to a Catholic school in Lancashire in the nineties. Discussing my vaginal woes is not in my DNA. It's the last thing I ever thought I'd be saying out loud and the very last thing I ever thought I'd write a book about. But you know what? Bollocks to it. We can name these conditions without the sky falling in. And we have to, because, if we don't, how will we ever shake off the shame so firmly attached to them? How will we ever get the research or the treatments we deserve? We're just setting up another generation to suffer in silence.

Our bodies are amazing, but we're not superhuman. We're sold a dream of 'bouncing back' when, in reality, the damage that can happen in pregnancy and childbirth can be enduring, debilitating even. Sometimes we feel it straight away. Sometimes it shows up years later. Rarely is it properly discussed or understood. But I'm writing this book because I want you to know that, when we find a way to say the unsayable, there is community, there is hope, we are stronger and our voices are louder.

I'll go first. I have pelvic organ prolapse. My pelvic organs fell out of place a couple of weeks after a gruelling second birth and ended up bulging into the wall of my vagina. I know. I had no idea it was possible either.

It turns out that your pelvic floor is made up of an

amazing group of muscles and tissues that form a sort of hammock at the base of your pelvis. Among other things, they support the pelvic organs (like the bladder, bowel and uterus); they help keep you continent by controlling the openings to the bladder and bowel; and they're important for sexual function too. But they can go wrong. They can become damaged, weak, overstretched or too tight – often during pregnancy and childbirth, as well as when your hormones change around menopause, or sometimes for other reasons like if you're overweight or have chronic constipation. When these muscles are not working as they should, there is a knock-on effect. And it's surprisingly common.

Researchers don't always agree, but it's estimated that one in three women have pelvic floor issues of some sort, making it more common than hay fever.[1] Let that sink in for a minute: one in three. Maybe, like me, it's prolapse, or maybe they leak wee or poo, while others will have pelvic pain, back pain or pain during sex. The umbrella term is 'pelvic floor dysfunction', though sometimes they're called disorders, and some lucky people will have a delightful collection of the above. That's around 10 million of us in the UK alone and, let's be honest, it's probably more, because so many of us don't report it.

Of course, everyone's experience will differ, and some symptoms are milder than others, but none of it should be taken lightly. Nobody wants to be left with wet knickers if they sneeze, cough or run; or to risk an 'accident' during their most intimate moments. They don't want to live with discomfort or chronic pain, or feel afraid to lift their children, or give up a job they love because they can't physically manage it. This is the thing about pelvic floor problems. They creep into every aspect of your life – parenting, work, fitness, body image, relationships – often on top of being an exhausted new mum and sometimes alongside other birth injuries. It's no wonder one study found that women with these conditions were three times more likely to have symptoms of depression.[2]

If you consider the scale and impact of all this, you'd think it would be common knowledge throughout our lives: that you'd learn about it in school, hear about it in the news and read about it in the pregnancy books. But you don't. You are, instead, side-swiped by this shocking thing that's happened to a part of your body you know virtually nothing about. Treatments are limited, information is limited, support is limited. You are on your own.

In 2018 I did something completely out of character: I decided to share my story on Instagram – anonymously at first – reaching out to anyone who might be able to relate or offer some quiet reassurance. I don't really know what I was expecting, except that I knew there must be others feeling the same way. I was right – total strangers understood perfectly and started talking about their own experiences. That's when I decided to do something even more out of character: I put my name on it. You can't smash taboos with a paper bag on your head, can you? Also, I'd just turned forty – if I couldn't own it now, when would I ever? I was writing about my wonky vagina in a public forum, and I was terrified. But then I was angry because here we all were, having these hushed conversations online, quietly suffering, confused and anxious; hiding away and blaming ourselves even though it happened through no fault of our own. I'm still angry, for lots of reasons.

Angry because what if it could be prevented? I came out of surgery after having a baby and a serious perineal tear, yet I had no idea that straining, lifting and everyday exertion could be the last straw for my pelvic floor. How could I? I barely knew what one was. What if I'd left hospital armed with that information? Would my postpartum recovery have been any different? What if I'd gone into hospital armed with that information? Would I have made different choices during the birth? Would I have acted differently through pregnancy? I know, it might have happened regardless . . . but I can't help but wonder.

Angry too because, when it does happen, some women spend years trying to persuade a doctor that things 'down there' aren't right. Or are greeted with a shrug and told, 'You've had a baby. What do you expect?' Worse than that, in 2020 an inquiry ordered by the UK government which looked at pelvic mesh implants found that women with prolapse or stress incontinence had sometimes suffered 'avoidable harm', their concerns dismissed as 'women's problems'.[3] It's another example of how we have so far to go when it comes to women's health; how not enough is known about conditions that only affect women; how the gender gap in health research is gaping; and how, in the words of Matt Hancock, the UK health secretary in 2021, 'For generations, women have lived with a health and care system that is mostly designed by men, for men.'[4]

That's assuming we even come forward to ask for help. Because how do you do that when you're too embarrassed to even mention it? I'm angry because society has taught us that anything to do with our vaginas is shameful and should be hidden away. We're talking centuries of shame – layer upon layer. It's a lot to unpick. And anyway, we would need to have the right words, which we don't. Don't get me wrong, I love a good euphemism, but research suggests that one in three of us still can't label the vulva on a simple diagram, let alone a urethra.[5] I'll admit I only learned in recent years that what most of us know as a vagina is a vulva. So let's clear this up right now: your vulva is the external genitals – all the bits on the outside.

I made a podcast to try to change things. A place where we could laugh, cry and cringe our way towards recovery or acceptance. A place where we could find trusted information and where stonkingly brave women – you'll meet some of them in this book – could share their stories. I cannot overstate the power in that, in knowing that you're not alone in the world and hearing others express your deepest, unspoken thoughts and fears.

I'm a radio producer by trade, so I was comfortable with the technical stuff. Less so with the speaking-about-my-vagina-in-public stuff. I'm still working on that. But the response has blown me away. Messages started coming in from around the world and they haven't stopped. Listeners have entrusted me with their own stories. They've told me how they're grieving for their former selves; how they feel aged and isolated; and how they're too embarrassed to discuss it with friends. But they've also told me how hearing from others has given them hope – that it's inspired them to be more open with loved ones, or that they've sought medical help after years of suffering in silence. One woman said she had cried tears of relief into a chicken pie; another, that she made her partner listen to every single episode! (Kudos to them.)

This book is for women of all ages who have found themselves with pelvic floors that have gone awry. It's also for their significant others and the people who love them and want to understand. It has grown out of my own experience as a woman and a mum, and you'll hear those words a lot, but I know that not everyone who experiences these issues will identify as a woman and, if that's you, I want you to know that you are also very welcome.

I'm not a medical expert, and you should absolutely seek out your own professional advice, but I do have a collection of rich narratives from the badass women I've had the privilege to meet. Strong women with tales that are as unique as they are universal. Women who have cried and laughed and screamed in the woods; asked themselves whether they would ever be normal again; battled to navigate the healthcare system; invented new treatments;

fought chronic pain; and hidden leaks from loved ones. Women who have gone through the wringer and come out the other side; who have gone on to have more babies; who have found sisterhood and friendship; who have embraced their 'feisty old crone'; and done it all with good humour and grace.

These voices need to be heard, and not just heard but amplified. Because if we want better treatment and research, more information and support, we have to find a way to talk about this. And what better time to do it than when conversations are beginning to open up about menopause, about periods, about gynaecological cancers and sexual health, about miscarriage and fertility treatment? I'm not saying you need to grab a megaphone and stand on your doorstep shouting it to the world, or make a podcast,

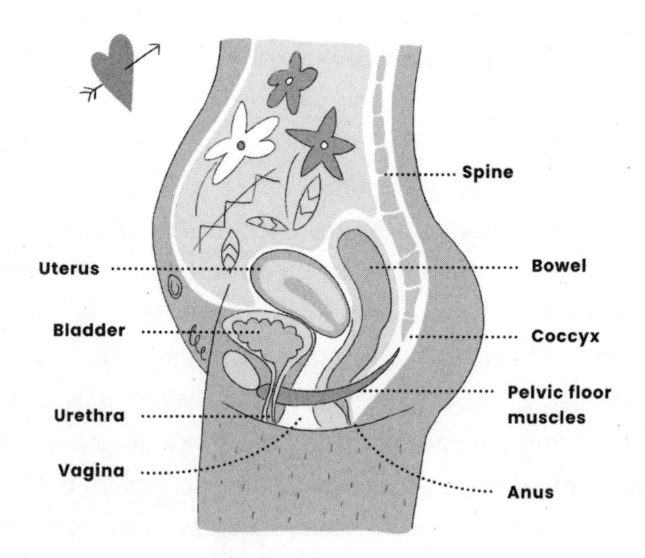

or reveal all on social media. But do bend someone's ear. I really think that's how we start to end the stigma.

I'm not going to tell you how to do your Kegels. I'm not even going to tell you that you have to do your Kegels. But by sharing these stories I want to show you that you are not alone, that there is hope and that, when we come together, we are stronger, and much harder to ignore.

The Pelvic Floor

- The pelvic floor is made up of muscles and tissues that form a sort of hammock across the base of the pelvis.
- It helps to keep the internal organs in their correct position and is important for bladder, bowel and sexual function. It also works with the abdominal muscles to help support the spine.
- The pelvic floor can become weak, overstretched, damaged or too tight, often (but not always) because of pregnancy and childbirth.
- It's estimated that one in three women experience problems with their pelvic floor – for example, incontinence, prolapse or pelvic pain.[6]
- These problems can be treated. Don't be embarrassed to talk to your GP.

CHAPTER 1

MY STORY

Let me take you back to March 2015. I'm thirty-six years old. It's the middle of the afternoon and I'm sitting half-naked on my bedroom floor with a make-up mirror in one hand and a phone in the other, wondering whether or not to call an ambulance.

I'd given birth to my son a couple of weeks earlier. He came crashing into the world, with his balled-up fists and white-blonde hair, almost exactly two years after his sister. It wasn't the easiest of births. I wasn't in great shape. I couldn't sit down without a pillow. But this? This was new – a sudden feeling that something was blocking my vagina, like I was losing a tampon. So I'm looking. And my heart is pounding because, if I'm honest, I don't really know what it's all supposed to look like, but it definitely isn't this. I google some words that describe what I see (I do not recommend that you do this!) and I eventually land on the term 'pelvic organ prolapse'. I mean, really? My insides are falling out? Saggy boobs and stretch marks – that's what I thought I'd be getting. Not this.

I didn't know that the pelvic floor muscles are supposed to keep your pelvic organs in place. Or that supporting the weight of a growing baby puts a lot of strain on them. Or that they stretch during childbirth and can become too weak or damaged to work properly. Or that, when that happens, one or more of those organs can slip out of place and into the vaginal wall. I didn't know that it can get worse over time, or that there is no reliable fix. I didn't know that it could change how you feel about your body, how you move, how you live your life. I didn't know that it could make you feel alone, broken, ashamed. I didn't know any of this, because no one ever talks about it.

Common symptoms of prolapse include a vaginal bulge or lump, discomfort, heaviness or dragging, bladder or bowel problems, or pain during sex, but it's hard to get a clear picture of how many people are affected. Not everyone with prolapse will experience symptoms, or at least not straight away; definitions vary; women are too embarrassed to report it; the research just isn't there. But the National Institute for Health and Care Excellence (NICE), which puts together the official health guidance for England, says that prevalence is 'high'. It says, when asked, 8.4 per cent of women reported feeling a bulge or lump, but that on examination, up to *50 per cent of all women* will have some degree of prolapse. And it says *one in ten* will eventually need surgery for it.[1]

It's widely agreed that this is a significant issue, not a rare condition that only affects a tiny section of society. And, while it's not life-threatening, it can seriously affect your physical well-being and quality of life. So it's kind of amazing that so few of us have heard about it before it happens. I was a second-time mum – you would think I'd have had a vague idea, but really, not a whisper.

My first child, my daughter, was born by elective caesarean after turning breech. Feet down. Legs crossed. We found out about her gymnastics on her due date and were advised that a C-section would be the safest option. So that was that. And thankfully it all went incredibly smoothly, but I had this sense that I'd cheated in some way because I hadn't tried for a vaginal birth, that my body had failed me, or maybe I hadn't given it a chance. I think I blamed the C-section for the breastfeeding difficulties and endless sleepless nights that nearly broke us. It sounds silly to me now, but it's how I felt. So when I got pregnant for a second time I was determined to have the beautiful vaginal birth promised by the pregnancy books and antenatal classes. I wanted to at least try for the unmedicated water birth and the candles, the carefully chosen playlist and the faster recovery. It didn't work out that way.

I'll spare you the blow-by-blow, but I didn't get anywhere near a birthing pool. It was a long labour with a lot of back pain and vomiting. Concern over my son's heart rate meant my waters were broken for me and, from then on, it was like someone had turned up the dial to full power. My body was pushing, violently, and I had no control. I was really scared. He must have been stuck because somewhere in the haze I agreed to an episiotomy. A cut, a last push and then he was out – fighting fit and raring to go, unlike his mum, who was a bit of a wreck. I had torn badly: a third-degree tear from the vagina, through the perineum and into the anal sphincter – the muscle that controls the anus. I was whisked off for surgery straight away.

In the UK, it's estimated that severe tears – third and fourth degree – happen in up to 6 per cent of first births.[2] They're known as obstetric and sphincter injuries (OASI) and are about as fun as they sound. They increase the risk of developing pelvic floor problems, and are known as a leading cause of bowel incontinence in women of reproductive age.[3,4] After surgery to repair them, most women recover fully, but up to four in ten will go on to have lasting complications.[5]

The charity Mothers with Anal Sphincter Injuries in Childbirth (MASIC) supports women with severe tears, which it says can have a 'devastating impact on quality of life'. It wants women to be told during pregnancy about the risk of having a serious tear.[6] I know not everyone will agree – some will see it as scaremongering – but, to me, it's just a sensible approach, because how can you make good birth choices if you don't have all the information to hand? How can you give yourself the best chance of recovery? If you have a hip operation, you're told there's a 1 per cent chance of infection afterwards;[7] if you have surgery for varicose veins, you're told there's a small risk of deep vein thrombosis (again, 1 per cent);[8] so why on earth aren't you warned about this?

It's important, too, because these tears are often missed at the time of delivery, meaning they're left unrepaired, which makes long-term problems even more likely.[9] Professor Michael Keighley is a retired colorectal surgeon who set up MASIC. I spoke to him during my research for this book and he told me, 'These injuries have a major impact on a woman's life within the family and in social society. If they're warned about it in pregnancy and it happens to them, they know they can go to their GP on the understanding that this isn't normal.' Women are not children. We can handle the truth. We shouldn't be left asking, 'Why did no one tell me?'

When I was told I had a third-degree tear, I had no clue what that meant. I knew it wasn't good, but only because the midwives were so sympathetic. I had no sense of the scale of the damage or what it might mean in the future. I remember lying in the operating theatre, deliriously quizzing the surgeon about his sewing skills, and still feeling like I'd done birth 'properly' this time around. Most people have a 'little tear' when they have a baby, don't they? A 'few' stitches? My son had exited via the correct orifice so how bad could it be? I thought I'd be back to myself in no time, and I didn't get much chance to dwell on it because now I was mum to a toddler and a newborn.

The problem with this lack of knowledge is that it leaves you vulnerable. Had I understood more about my own anatomy, had I known the tear made me more likely to develop a prolapse, would I have done more to protect myself? It wasn't like I was doing the cancan or anything, but maybe I wouldn't have strained on the loo or lifted my toddler – two things that put your pelvic floor muscles under stress and two things I did on the day things went south. After my caesarean, two years earlier, I knew that for the first six weeks I shouldn't drive or lift anything heavier than the baby. It didn't occur to me that a tear could be as serious.

I know prolapse can happen even if you have the smoothest of births, are waited on hand and foot, wrapped in cotton wool and are able to sleep for eight hours every night. It can happen if you've never had a vaginal birth and even if you've never had a baby. Nevertheless, I can't help feeling that an awareness of the state I was in might have helped to prevent it. But it just wasn't part of any conversation I'd heard around birth. Not in the books, not in the classes, not at medical appointments, not from other mums, not anywhere.

I'm not alone in this. In 2021 more than 3000 mums in the UK and US responded to a survey about postpartum recovery by MUTU System, a pre- and postnatal fitness app.[10] The vast majority (91 per cent) did not feel they were given enough advice during pregnancy. We are told what to pack in our hospital bags and how to write a birth plan, but very little about how to heal afterwards. It's important to say that every year millions of women around the world give birth without any problems, but we still need a realistic idea of what our bodies go through and, crucially, what will give us the best chance of recovery. We can do better. We have to do better, because it has a huge impact on people's lives.

When I realized I had a prolapse, I thought, 'I'll just get it fixed. There's bound to be a way to put everything back where it was before, right?' But it's not as simple as that. Like with other pelvic floor problems, there is no magic pill. Surgical options are limited (serious operations which carry risks and can be short-lived); pelvic health physiotherapy can help, but it isn't a 'cure'; and, beyond that, it's about managing the symptoms – incontinence, pain or discomfort; some people really suffer, others less so. For me, there was a constant feeling of heaviness, like I was sitting on a doorknob. I still feel a bulge, sometimes more than others. At its worst it's uncomfortable and annoying, like wearing underwear that's two sizes too small. Periods are a mission because neither tampons nor menstrual cups will stay in, and toileting is not what it was – I can't always empty my bowels fully.

Then there are the lifestyle constraints. For years, the medical advice has been to stay away from things that put a lot of pressure on your pelvic floor. It makes sense – you really don't want this to get worse if you can help it, but when you consider what this guidance means in daily life, you'll see how limiting it can be. You're told to avoid high-impact exercise like running or anything that involves jumping; avoid being overweight (not so easy when you are avoiding exercise); avoid heavy lifting (tricky when you're laden with babies, toddlers, car seats and buggies); and, while you're at it, avoid standing for long periods of time. I did what I was told. I'm quite attached to my pelvic organs, and I was terrified that one wrong move would see me waving goodbye to them for good. I call this 'The Fear'.

The trouble with The Fear is that it puts every single

action through a filter of anxiety. If I do this, will it make things worse? Never mind running a marathon or climbing a mountain, what about pushing a buggy, carrying your baby in a sling, lifting the groceries, digging the weeds, doing your job, living your life? Before I had children I was fit. Not Olympic-level fit, but I played a bit of netball, I could jog around the park and attempt a terrible cartwheel on a beach. Now, I was afraid of movement. I said goodbye to the desire to return to the active person I was and resigned myself to lifelong restrictions. I stopped dancing around the kitchen with my kids and chasing after them on their scooters. I stopped lifting them or anything else unless it was absolutely necessary, and I found myself telling them that 'Mummy isn't strong' or 'Mummy can't do that'. What sort of role modelling is that for the next generation? It made me really sad. It's not who I was. It's not who I am.

This is the problem with such broad-brush advice. It's well intended, but it doesn't take into account what your lifestyle is like or the fact that everyone is different. Nor does it recommend alternative ways to stay active. When you're limited in this way, it's really hard to stay fit, to stay healthy. And it's short-sighted. We are telling all adults they should be exercising every day, apart from this whole group of women who are now storing up even more health problems for the future. As we'll hear, that narrative is slowly changing, but more research is needed so that we can start to give women proper advice about how to move, instead of telling them to just . . . stop.

My story is absolutely not one of endless doom and gloom. I want you to know that now. Seven years on, I lift my kids, I dance around the kitchen, I even run. But, for a long time, my prolapse quietly consumed me and I really struggled to understand exactly what it was, what it meant, what I should or shouldn't do about it and what the future might look like. It's not like there was a national helpline or a support group or a UK charity for mums with fallen organs. And the internet was full of conflicting advice, turning up more lists of exercises to avoid, telling me I was sitting incorrectly, eating incorrectly, even breathing incorrectly. You can cure it. You can't cure it. Kegels are the answer, but also Kegels could make it worse. And, by the way, when menopause hits, it's pretty much game over. It was just so confusing. In trying to answer these questions I ended up in a bleak rabbit hole of online forums with women who themselves were sharing their lowest moments with strangers because they didn't feel able to turn to anyone else. This was how it was; I was lost.

For the next three years I got on with the not-so-small task of being a working mum-of-two, quietly managing my symptoms and living with The Fear. What else was I going to do? We're so programmed to think that this is a 'normal' part of having children that, even as I type, I'm questioning whether I'm making a big deal out of nothing. I know I have a lot to be thankful for – healthy kids, a supportive partner, a comfortable life – but pelvic floor problems *are* a big deal, and in lots of different ways. I really want to try to get across the enduring impact they can have.

Women often write and tell me how they can't run any more, or dance or garden without discomfort. How they're in too much pain to sway their baby to sleep or that they can't bend down to bathe their child without leaking. Sometimes they sit on bin bags in the car to avoid soiling the seat. Sometimes they avoid leaving the house at all. They tell me their pelvic floor problems are an 'invisible disability' with a 'seismic' impact and that they're shocked, ashamed and too embarrassed to talk about any of it. It's not OK. It's why I decided to make the podcast.

I wanted it to be a place where you *could* talk about it. Where you could hear from other women in their own words and know that you were not alone. And I knew it had to begin with my own story, but when I tell you that articulating that was hard, it really was. It's one thing sharing your innermost thoughts about your innermost parts on an Instagram post, but actually saying them out loud is something else entirely. I had never done that before. I couldn't just pick up a microphone and pour my heart out. I needed some help.

Cath is my best friend. I feel like I'm about eight years old saying that, but it's true. We met at school thirty years ago when she rocked a hot pink shell suit and I wore my fringe clipped back in a bump (or was it a pouf?). We sneaked into our first pubs together, sat exams, travelled abroad, met boyfriends, got married and had babies. She's the perfect person to give me a kick up the ass because there's nothing this woman does not know about me. And yet when it came to recording that first episode, I was so nervous on the drive to her house that my palms were sweating.

When I arrived, she was sweeping out a newly plastered kitchen wearing her husband's grey joggers. There was dust everywhere and she was telling me all about the renovation plans, but I wasn't really taking it in. There was too much going on in my head. Even if I got past the embarrassment of sharing my issues in all their glory, I wasn't sure I would be able to hold it together emotionally. We borrowed the builder's kettle, made a brew and then I turned down a Hob-nob, which, if you know me, tells you everything. We settled down on the floor in the back bedroom, and I propped up my phone against a cushion and pressed record.

I told Cath that pelvic floor problems are life-changing. That they affect everything about who you are, how you live your life and how you parent. That they make you question every move in case things get worse. And that you blame yourself because maybe you should have known, should have made better choices, should have done more Kegels. I told her how I felt like I would never be the mum I imagined I would be (that's the bit that gets me every time), that I thought I'd never chase my kids on the beach, that there would be no piggyback rides, that I just wouldn't be me anymore.

I said I was angry that so many women were living with these conditions in isolation because no one ever talks about them. And I felt like these problems might sometimes be avoided, but neither the information nor the support was there. I explained how hearing other women's experiences was helping me to come to terms with mine, and then Cath gently teased me about my struggle to use anatomical terms. 'Stop saying fanny,' she said. She's not wrong. That's been a journey in itself.

This all happened in the days before Covid. In the days when you could hug people without giving it a second thought. Thank goodness. I needed one after that.

Pelvic Organ Prolapse (Vaginal Prolapse)

- Pelvic organ prolapse (POP) is when one or more of the organs in the pelvis (for example, the bladder, bowel or uterus) slips down from its normal position and bulges into the vagina.
- It happens when the muscles and connective tissues of the pelvic floor are overstretched, weakened or damaged, and can no longer support the pelvic organs.
- Symptoms include a feeling of bulging, heaviness or dragging, incontinence, pelvic pain or discomfort during sex.
- With the right guidance, symptoms can be improved with lifestyle changes, pelvic floor rehabilitation, pessaries (vaginal inserts that help to hold everything up) or sometimes surgery.

- If you have symptoms, ask your GP for a referral to a pelvic health physiotherapist for diagnosis and treatment.
- It's not your fault. It's nothing to be ashamed about. You are not alone.

CHAPTER 2

AINSLEY

(THE DOCTOR WILL SEE YOU NOW)

Getting treatment for your pelvic floor problems is a lottery. There's no other word for it. It's a game of chance that depends on where you live, who the gatekeepers are and, like so many things, whether you're in a position to pay for it. You could say my numbers came up because, when I discovered my prolapse, two weeks after my son was born, I was still under the care of a midwife. So once the panic subsided and I decided not to call an ambulance, I had someone to turn to. I was still worried, but, I think you'll agree, I wore it well:

27 Mar 2015, 15:31

Hiya. Prepare for TMI. I'm wondering if I might have a bit of a problem down below...maybe prolapse and piles? Just not sure how urgent it might be? Should I be trying for a doc appointment or wait to see you on Mon? Sorry! Helen

The midwife advised me to see my GP, so I made the call and took the first appointment, a fortnight away. I spent the next fourteen days walking on eggshells, afraid to lift anything other than my newborn, afraid to even consider what the future might look like. I was looking for an explanation and hoping for a fix, or at least some reassurance. But when I dragged my sorry body (and my baby) to the surgery, still in a state of shock over the state of my nethers, the doctor did not seem to share my concern. She examined me briefly and wearily, confirmed prolapse (not piles) and sent me away with a shoulder shrug and the promise of a referral letter, which hadn't materialized when I called a week later. Knowing what I know now, I can almost understand this indifference. I was in emergency mode, but she sees new mums like me day in, day out – women who are struggling with unspoken injuries that they don't understand and that nobody seems interested in, conditions that may not be life-threatening, but are certainly life-changing. I see now that our perspectives were very different, but I felt so let down. It's the only time in my life I have changed GP. I couldn't face seeing her again.

That was my experience in 2015. Looking back, I think it could have been worse. After I chased up the NHS referral, I was seen, within months, by a urogynaecologist. A year later I had a few sessions with a pelvic health physiotherapist. So I had a level of support, but I hear regularly from women who've plucked up the courage to ask their GP for help, only to be sent away – sometimes with a referral, but often with just a leaflet or with nothing at all. 'This is normal when you have babies' is the message they're given, and sometimes with those exact words. They're told, 'It's the price of having children,' or simply, 'Women's bodies are badly designed,' which honestly beggars belief. And it leaves them feeling foolish and ashamed, because why hadn't they realized this was how it was? And if they had, could they have done something to prevent it?

Six weeks after her first son was born, Ainsley Howard got her mirror out. She had noticed a heaviness around her pelvis since the birth, and incontinence too, but she had so many other aches and pains through pregnancy and in the early weeks of motherhood that she thought it must be part and parcel of it. When she finally braved a look and realized things weren't right, she went to see her GP. 'It's normal,' she was told. 'Come back in three months if things don't improve.' Ainsley went away. She tried to accept it, but things didn't improve. So she returned three months later, with much the same result: 'They kind of just said, "Well, that's it." You know? "You've got a prolapse." They said they'd seen worse. And just sent me on my way. So I mean, what do you do with that information?'

Ainsley lives in Manchester and is an actor – you might know her from the British comedy drama *Mount Pleasant* or as the voice of Fizzy Izzy in the kids' TV series *Digby Dragon*. She was also the first woman to share her story on the podcast. I met her through a mutual friend and jumped for joy (metaphorically) when she agreed to speak to me, because finding and then persuading people to talk publicly about their pelvic floor problems is no easy task. It's not something people tend to advertise, and asking for a status update on someone's vagina is just not the done thing. Such is the shame and secrecy, people start to imagine who might hear it and, understandably, what the personal or professional impact might be. It really is an incredibly brave thing to do. I wish it wasn't and I hope it won't always be this way, but I never underestimate it.

I know it wasn't an easy decision for Ainsley to appear on the podcast, but from our very first conversation, she understood what I was trying to do and she wanted to help. If speaking about her experience made it easier for the next person or brought comfort to someone who was struggling, then it was worth it. She would do it. So I was very grateful to find myself sitting in her living room one winter's evening, curtains drawn, cup of tea in hand and slightly in awe of this gorgeous young mum who was sharing her experience so candidly with someone she had only just met. Not to mention the fact that she was heavily pregnant – just days away, as it turned out, from giving birth to her second son.

Like so many of us, Ainsley had never heard of pelvic organ prolapse until she was told she had one. She was shocked, but then given no help to manage it. And while the heaviness or 'dragging' feeling she'd been experiencing was improving with time, the incontinence wasn't. It was getting worse. 'You end up putting a pad on and then thinking that's normal,' she told me, 'but then I'm thinking, I'm thirty-six. I don't want to wear a pad in case I sneeze or cough. I don't feel ready for that yet!'

Urinary incontinence is defined by the International Continence Society as 'the involuntary loss of urine'.[1] Again, it's hard to know how many women are affected, because it depends on how you define it, who you ask and how you measure it. And you can add to that the embarrassment factor, which stops people from reporting it in the first place. But most studies agree that somewhere between 25 and 45 per cent of women experience urinary incontinence to some degree.[2] It's twice as common in women as men.[3] And there's a whole list of things that make it more likely, including pregnancy, childbirth and increasing age, thanks to the hormonal changes that come with menopause.[4]

There are different types of incontinence too. The ones you're most likely to hear about are stress incontinence, where you leak if you cough, laugh, sneeze or jump; and urge incontinence, where you suddenly need the toilet and just can't hang on. Some people have the joys of both. Bar the occasional blip, and despite my pelvic floor issues, I am not affected by it. I don't know why. But I do know that, for those who are, it impacts their quality of life in a very real way. It can lead to rashes, ulcers and urinary tract infections. And research shows that incontinence is associated with poor body image and low self-esteem, especially when it's been going on for a long time.[5] When women were asked, they spoke about the chore of constantly using pads, the discomfort of feeling damp, the fear of smelling bad and a feeling of being unclean or inadequate. I mean, of course it's going to affect how you feel about yourself.

Ainsley told me it was tough. She expected her body to change after giving birth, but not like this: 'Sometimes, if I'm out with friends and I start laughing, I wet myself. And for a split couple of seconds, I'm relieved, like "Thank God I put a pad on." And then if I forget to put a pad on, I've got wet knickers and I've not got anywhere to go. And then I'm in the middle of town or at a meeting or something and just feel like . . . I don't know. Not ashamed but just . . . down, fed up, a bit miserable about it. But then, there's never enough time to really dwell on it because that's it, you're a mum now, and someone else is first and foremost.'

I guarantee that there are women around you right now who've found their own ways of coping with the leaks and lumps they've been told are 'normal'. They're wearing pads and dark clothes, limiting their fluid intake, avoiding exercise and intimacy. They're mapping out the nearest toilets, making jokes about trampolines and crossing their legs when they sneeze – all because of an ingrained perception that these conditions should be accepted as part of motherhood. But while this approach might help to mask the problem, in no way does it address it. In fact it's more likely to lead to further health problems because, you know, not exercising or drinking enough isn't a great way to stay fit and well.

There's no quick fix for incontinence (you're going to

hear me say this a lot), but treatments are available. For example, there's good evidence that two-thirds of women will see improvement or even cure with pelvic floor muscle training – where you're assessed and then taught how to squeeze and relax the pelvic floor to make the muscles stronger, to build endurance or coach them to relax.[6] Yes, it's Kegels, but it can also include stretching and breathing exercises, strength training and more. You might also be advised to make lifestyle changes like cutting down on caffeine or losing weight, and medicines can be prescribed, as can non-surgical interventions like bladder injections. For some people, conversations with surgeons will have to take place. It's a process, but there are options, once you get the support you need.

When Ainsley's son was one, she went back to the GP for a third time and was referred for physiotherapy. Over several sessions, she was given a programme of exercise, recommended a pelvic floor app and given tips and strategies to help manage the incontinence. She says it really helped. She was starting to get somewhere. But it had taken a year and three visits to the doctor to get the ball rolling, and that was before Covid happened. I've heard from women since who've waited two, even three, years for NHS treatment.

There's no doubt in my mind that we are failing women by leaving them for so long without the help and information they need, often at such a vulnerable time in their lives. And you can put this in the context of a wider problem. Since the start of the Covid pandemic, and across the board, waiting lists for tests, surgery and routine treatment have hit record highs.[7] Fair enough, you might think. But now consider that in that time, in England, the waiting list for gynaecology has gone up by more than 60 per cent – the sharpest increase of all medical specialities.[8] It's a list that was growing even before the pandemic. As I write, there are more than half a million names on it, and 25,000 of them will wait a year or more for care. All of them experiencing symptoms that stop them from living a full life. It's about priorities, and it's an issue that was raised in April 2022 by the Royal College of Obstetricians and Gynaecologists (RCOG). In a statement, the RCOG president, Dr Edward Morris, said: 'We believe the reason gynaecology waiting lists have seen the biggest growth is because time and again we see women's health consistently deprioritized and overlooked. At its core it is gender bias and it's reflective of society as a whole. Women are being let down and change is urgently needed.'[9] It's something else we need to talk about. And we will.

As for getting on to a waiting list in the first place, like with so many NHS services, there are countrywide variations in how to access care. It's honestly taken me until now to almost get my head around it. The GP can be a good first port of call, but it's not necessarily the only way to get specialist help. Depending on where you live, you might also get a referral from your midwife, obstetrician or health visitor. In some areas you can self-refer. Then you might be seen by a physiotherapist or a consultant or a specialist nurse.

You could be seen in person or offered a remote assessment. You could even be invited to join a group class. And if you need further treatment, there are a multitude of routes you might then take. The whole thing can happen in weeks, or it can take months, or, as we've heard, years. It's not an easy system to navigate and, unfortunately, you're still at risk of bumping into ill-informed or old-fashioned attitudes. It shouldn't happen, but sometimes it does. One woman told me she was 'fobbed off' by a doctor several months after her daughter was born, despite the fact that she couldn't walk without leaking, and despite being a doctor herself. It took a second opinion to get the help she needed. Another was asked, 'Is it really the end of the world if you can't go running or spinning anymore?' Well, it might be, if that's how you maintain your mental health.

Given these obstacles, it's not surprising that some women choose to pay for private treatment, but if we take physiotherapy as an example, where one appointment can cost £100 or more, it's simply not an option for everyone. Some will be able to claim on their medical insurance, but even that's less straightforward than you'd think. In 2021 the insurance firm Aviva was taken to task on social media after a patient with incontinence was refused payment for physiotherapy. The reason she was given at the time was that she'd had a baby, so it was seen as a consequence of choice. Her husband's football-related knee injury though? That was covered. When the physio-led campaign group Pelvic Roar got involved, Aviva said the refusal wasn't, in fact, about lifestyle choice, and that its policy was consistent with other providers, but it reversed the decision and paid out for the claim.[10] It's since changed its terms and conditions so that incontinence after childbirth *is* covered, which is a good thing, but this was far from an isolated case. Several women told me they'd had a similar experience with other insurance firms. One said that she had to fight to get her physiotherapy covered, comparing it with a claim she'd made previously for an ankle ligament injury. 'I asked the manager, "What made my ankle eligible and my vagina not?" He apologized profusely and immediately authorized the sessions.'

The thing is, you shouldn't have to make a manager squirm, or struggle on for years, or get a PhD in NHS pathways to get the help you need. And you don't have to look far to find somewhere that gives pelvic health a higher priority. France has long been held up as an example of best practice, a panacea for broken 'bits', if you like. And that's because, for decades, anyone who's just had a baby has been given a minimum of ten sessions of physio to 're-educate' their pelvic floor. State-funded since 1985, *La rééducation périnéale* starts six to eight weeks after birth to help prevent and treat pelvic floor dysfunction. It's standard practice. Free of charge. You leave hospital with the prescription. Recent changes mean that, in theory, it's now only for those with symptoms, but as one French physiotherapist pointed out to me, 'Who doesn't have symptoms after having a baby?' So it's still very much the norm.

A listener in France, Emmy, rolled her eyes with a smile when I asked her about this. She told me that nobody there even talks about *La rééducation* because it's so commonplace. You go twice a week for five weeks to see a physio or a specialist midwife (*sage-femme*), and they help you with your pelvic floor exercises using hands-on therapy and pelvic floor gadgets (we'll get to that). After that, there are usually another ten sessions to help rehabilitate your abdominal muscles, which *I* think sounds incredible. But she also pointed out that it's a one-size-fits-all affair, which is fine for many women, but starts to fall down if your situation is even remotely complex. And then there's the lingering focus on rehabilitation for the sake of your sex life or, more specifically, your 'husband's' sex life, which puts a slightly different slant on the whole thing, so she doesn't think it should be placed on a pedestal.

For all its flaws, having a universal system for pelvic floor rehabilitation makes sense to me, because why wouldn't you try to catch these issues early? Even if it's not the answer for everyone, it's going to help new mums to understand what their bodies have been through, where to access tools and resources, what's 'normal' and what's not. I really think, too, that anything that makes pelvic health an everyday conversation, something you can talk openly about, should be celebrated, because, ultimately, that's what will see off the stigma that can prevent women from even asking for help in the first place.

There have been calls for the UK to adopt the French

approach, but recently published health guidelines suggest that there isn't enough evidence to support offering it to everyone or to show that it's 'cost effective', so it's unlikely to happen, or at least not anytime soon.[11,12] The landscape is shifting though. NHS England has acknowledged that it needs to do more when it comes to preventing and treating pelvic floor issues. In 2019, it promised to make it easier for new mums to get pelvic health physiotherapy as well as to improve pelvic health care more generally.[13] And, as a result, it's investing in fourteen areas of the country, where specialist doctors, midwives and physios are working along-side each other, and where you should be able to self-refer if you're pregnant or a new mum.[14] It's funding training, as well as paying for new resources to help women get the information they so badly need. And by 2024, the idea is to expand all of that so that it's available right across the country.

So a slow change is coming, and there's money behind it, as well as this raft of new guidelines on the prevention and non-surgical management of pelvic floor dysfunction.[15] They're going to crop up a few times in the book so it's worth explaining that these are evidence-based recommendations for health and care in England. They're the first of their kind, published by NICE in 2021, to try to prevent pelvic floor dysfunction, raise awareness and minimize the use of surgery.[16] It's all very welcome, but we're not there yet. In the UK, there are currently not enough pelvic health physiotherapists to meet the need. And when I say there aren't enough, some areas don't have any. Not a single one. In 2020 researchers looked at what it would take to offer pelvic floor training for every woman with symptoms of prolapse – just prolapse, forget about all the other stuff for a minute – and they estimated that for every specialist physiotherapist in the UK, there were more than 2500 women in need of help.[17] There are also historical challenges around recruitment to a specialism that has long been overlooked. For example, pelvic health is not even on the curriculum for physiotherapy students. If they're taught it at all, it's for a couple of hours over the entire three-year course. And, by the way, it's not taught consistently to trainee nurses, doctors or midwives either.[18] You can see how getting any treatment at all can sometimes feel like an accomplishment in itself.

Five sessions with a physio got me a decent idea of how to do a pelvic floor squeeze (it's not as simple as you might think) and an understanding ear, which mattered a lot, because who else could I talk to, really? Similarly for Ainsley, physio set her on the right track, and that was important, not least because she was soon pregnant for a second time . . . and she was worried about her prolapse: 'I was really quite frightened about it. Even though the doctors said it was mild. I didn't want it to get worse.'

This is a huge concern for women with pelvic floor problems, especially if they had a difficult birth the first time around. 'Will having another baby make everything worse?' is the million-dollar question. And although research suggests that, statistically, symptoms are *un*likely to worsen with a

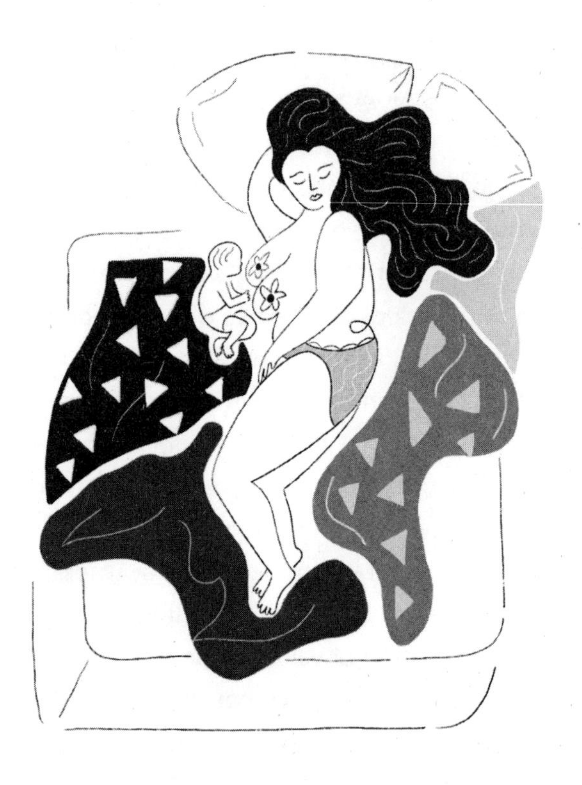

second delivery (vaginal or caesarean), in reality, there are no easy options.[19,20] It's going to depend on your starting point, your history, the birth itself and your recovery. It's one to discuss with your healthcare provider.

Clare Bourne is a pelvic health physiotherapist (and an Instagram queen in the world of subpar vaginas) who has a prolapse herself and went on to have a second vaginal birth. Despite all her expertise, even she was worried about doing it again. But when I spoke to her for the podcast, she told me that knowing she had recovered *once* to a point where she was symptom-free, gave her the confidence to go for it again: 'I thought, "Even if I'm more symptomatic for the first year, I know I still recovered much better in the second year, when maybe I was getting more sleep and had a bit more time to think about myself" and I think that lived experience has helped me to be a bit more relaxed and take the rough days as they come.'

Clare said that staying strong during pregnancy and following a postpartum fitness programme helped her to a point where, two years later, she's symptom-free most days. Her advice is to flag it as early as possible if you're worried, so you can get the information you need to make the best decision for you.

When Ainsley found out she was pregnant for a second time, she was set on having a caesarean. It felt to her like a safer bet. But after speaking to her consultant and weighing up the risks, she decided to try for another vaginal birth, and did everything she could to prepare for it. Alongside the physiotherapy, she practised yoga and says that, for her, studying hypnobirthing really helped too: 'I started thinking I don't have to be frightened. I can embrace it. I can strengthen my mind in a positive way to not be fearful and really just focus on getting my baby out safely, rather than what my prolapse is going to be like at the end of this.'

Ainsley delivered her second little boy just a few days after we recorded the podcast. She told me it all happened very quickly but that it went really well and that having another baby didn't make her pelvic floor problems any worse. Like so many of us, she still has good days and bad, but now she at least knows what she can do to help herself and where to go for support.

I hear stories like Ainsley's all the time – women who agonize over whether to put their pelvic floors through it all over again. Some decide not to, some opt for a caesarean, while others go for a vaginal delivery. I have yet to hear from anyone who has regretted their decision. What is clear though, is that women don't always feel supported or well informed in these choices. They shouldn't be left in the dark to the point where they're hunting me down on social media to ask whether they should request a caesarean (or even if they're allowed to), just like they shouldn't be waiting for months or years to be offered specialist help, or muddling through by themselves because they've been told it's 'normal' to leak, or to be in pain, or to live a restricted life. Getting basic care shouldn't be a lottery.

Urinary Incontinence

- Urinary incontinence can be defined as 'the involuntary loss of urine'.[21]
- There are two main types: stress incontinence, where you leak with exertion (for example, when you cough, sneeze or jump) and urgency (or urge) incontinence, where you suddenly need to wee and you can't hold

on. Mixed incontinence is when you have symptoms of both.

- Urinary incontinence is known to be a common problem, thought to affect between 25 and 45 per cent of women.[22]
- There's evidence that two-thirds of women (67 per cent) will see improvement or even cure with pelvic floor muscle training.[23]
- If you have symptoms, ask your GP for a referral to a pelvic health physiotherapist for diagnosis and treatment.

CHAPTER 3

PEACE

(EDUCATION, EDUCATION, EDUCATION)

It's true that, until a few years ago, I didn't really know what a vulva was. I used 'vagina' or 'fanny' as a catch-all term, but only when absolutely necessary. And I spent approximately zero minutes giving it any thought at all. I mean, if I gave you a diagram of the vulva (the external female genitalia), would you know where to find a labia, clitoris or urethra? Don't feel bad if the answer is no, because you are far, far from alone.

In March 2021 a group of gynaecologists handed out questionnaires in waiting rooms at a UK hospital, not just to patients but to their friends and families too. Participants were asked to label the different parts of the vulva in their own words. They didn't have to use the correct anatomical language – terms like 'peehole' (urethra) and 'bumhole' (anus) were enough – but, of those who gave it a go, only 9 per cent got all the structures correct. Nearly half left it blank. Maybe you're not surprised by that. As I say, until recently, I wouldn't have done any better. But then they were asked, 'How many holes does a woman have in her private parts?' and fewer than half (just 46 per cent) knew the right answer which, to avoid confusion, is three.[1]

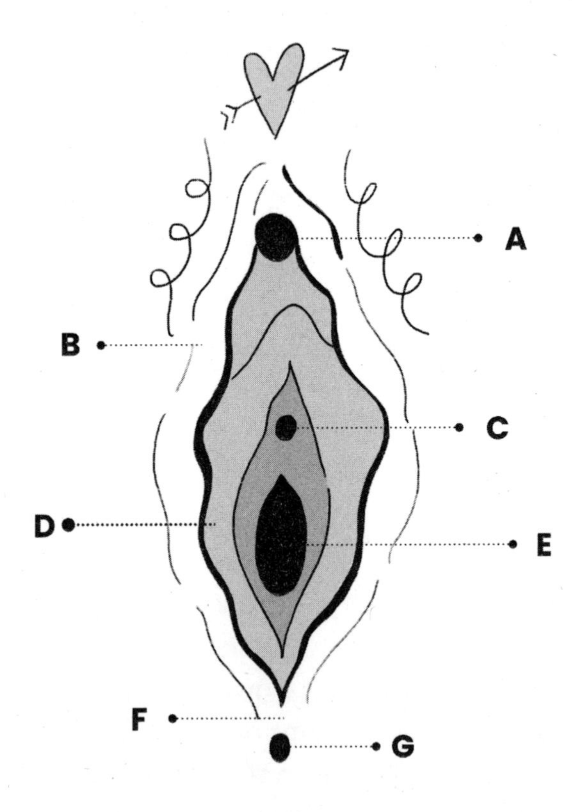

A: clitoris, B: labia majora, C: urethra, D: labia minora, E: vagina, F: perineum, G: anus

The research, published in the *International Urogynecology Journal,* was carried out because doctors were concerned about the number of patients they saw in gynae clinics who were confused about the nature of their problems. If people didn't know the basics, how could they make decisions about treatment? How could they give informed consent? With that in mind, they also looked at people's understanding of pelvic organ prolapse in comparison with other medical conditions. Most understood what stroke and diabetes were, but only half had even heard of prolapse. Dr Stephanie Shoop-Worrall is an epidemiologist at the University of Manchester and was involved in the study. She told the *Guardian* newspaper: 'If a doctor is going to examine you, or suggest any kind of treatment plan, you need to fully understand what's going to happen, and the risks and benefits, to be able to give permission. If people are coming in for their hospital appointment and not understanding basic anatomy, or what's even wrong with them, how can they properly consent to treatment?'[2]

It's not the first time our knowledge has been tested and found wanting. The Eve Appeal, a gynaecological cancer research charity, has been asking people to identify the different parts of the female genital anatomy in its surveys since 2014. It says things have improved a bit, but that one in three women is still unable to label the vulva on a diagram, often getting it mixed up with the vagina. Speaking to the *i* newspaper in 2022, the charity's CEO Athena Lamnisos said: 'The picture is pretty dismaying. If you don't know what's going on between your legs and inside your pelvis, and you don't know your own normal, you can't recognize when something isn't normal for you and seek medical help.'[3]

That's the danger, isn't it? If you don't know what's there, how do you know when things aren't OK? And if we're talking about cancer specifically, it's about as serious as it gets, because it's a fact that early diagnosis and treatment can save lives.

We've ended up in a situation where we're so clueless about our bodies that we're putting them at risk. And, even if we know the correct words, we can't bring ourselves to use them. You only have to listen to the first episode of the podcast to hear me squirming as I try to talk about my prolapse. And I'm not just talking about vaginas and vulvas here, but anything even remotely related to our pelvic anatomy. Julie Cornish is a consultant colorectal surgeon at the University Hospital of Wales, Cardiff. When I spoke to her, she explained how avoiding the correct terms can lead to unnecessary distress and delays in treatment. For example, she says that patients with bowel incontinence are sometimes too embarrassed to say that to a doctor. Instead they might say they have 'diarrhoea' – a change in bowel habits which can lead to them being treated as an urgent suspected cancer case. So they're referred to the wrong service for tests and, when they're eventually given the all-clear, they're right back where they started. 'And the woman goes, "Well, I wasn't asking if I had cancer, what I was asking is can you help with my bowel problems?"'

Language matters. And not just in the doctor's office. Because the other thing that happens when we use the wrong words is that it reinforces the shame around these parts of our bodies. I'm not leading the charge against euphemisms here – we've spent several lifetimes cultivating a list as long as your arm and the world would be a poorer place without it – but the danger with *relying* on these cute, ugly or sometimes totally bizarre names is that it sends a message that our genitals are unmentionable, or something to be horrified by, or that they should be hidden, ridiculed or covered up with a more acceptable word. It's a message that amplifies the stigma and can affect the way we view our bodies, relationships or intimacy. And it's a message that is being drilled into all of us all of the time, even without us realizing. Like when I used an auto-captioning service for a social media video and it censored the word 'vagina'. It really made me doubt myself. A handful of carefully placed asterisks made me question whether it *was* actually OK. *Should* I be exposing people, without warning, to this war-head of a word?

It's not easy. Most of us grew up with euphemisms as the go-to for our private parts and, as parents, that's a hard habit to break. It's awkward. It's uncomfortable. I confess I spent the first few years of my children's lives avoiding using any words at all. I have no idea how I managed to do that. But in making the podcast I've come to realize that if I want them to grow up feeling positive about their bodies and empowered to ask questions or seek help, I need to give them the language to do it. It shouldn't be a big deal – it certainly isn't for them – and it's important because, if we don't have the basics down, how will we ever be prepared when things don't go to plan? And, as we know, things don't always go to plan.

When Peace Bailey experienced night-time incontinence after childbirth she, like so many of us, was completely *un*prepared: 'I knew nothing, honestly, and, especially as I'm coming from an African background, there's no way my mother would have talked to me about that. If you heard the talk she had with me about the birds and bees you'd be horrified! So there's no way she would have explained the pelvic floor to me. I'm not even sure that she knows what it is herself, because it's just one of those things that would be too taboo, too private, and just a "Figure it out on your own" kind of thing.'

Peace was born in Rwanda, grew up in the UK and moved to Spain in 2019. I got in touch with her when I saw that she had quietly acknowledged her incontinence on Instagram. Among the technicolour posts about her new life in the sun, about parenting and body positivity, this one really stood out for its brutal honesty. 'Labour did a number on me,' it began, 'both times.' I asked her if she would speak to me about it on the podcast and she said she was happy to share. She's eloquent and thoughtful. And when we got to record, remotely, during the Covid lockdown, she told me that, after two births and two perineal tears, she was already struggling with her pelvic floor, but wetting the bed after her youngest son was born – that was the real wake-up call:

> It's something I never expected to happen to me. I never expected to wake up one morning and realize I've wet the bed, or wake up at night even, and have to quickly figure

> out how I'm going to hide this from my husband. Because how do I explain this? I don't even remember if I was able to go back to sleep because I was embarrassed. I couldn't even go in the shower cos it was like three or four in the morning. So I had to crawl back into bed trying to figure out what just happened. How is this happening to me? I'm thirty-four years old. What is this?

When it kept happening, Peace told her husband what was going on and, of course, he was hugely supportive. But she still felt alone because she didn't know what to do about it, and she didn't know who she could talk to. She eventually confided in a doctor friend, who was reassuring and sent some videos about pelvic floor exercises, but she struggled to understand how she was supposed to train these muscles that she couldn't see, and that she barely knew existed. I can relate to this. When you're going from a standing start, even the best video tutorial in the world is going to leave you scratching your head or, more likely (and incorrectly), clenching your bum. Peace just couldn't get to grips with it, so she put it to the bottom of her to-do list.

After months of hoping things would get better on their own, Peace started to realize they wouldn't. She wanted a functioning body. She wanted to be stronger, not just for now but for the future too. So she started pelvic floor training consistently – following the videos as best she could, and exercising more in general. She said it really helped – the accidents were happening less and less. Reflecting back,

Peace told me she wished she had acted sooner. Had she understood from the start what was happening, had she felt able to talk more openly about it, maybe she wouldn't have been blindsided by it. Maybe she wouldn't have suffered in silence: 'I think part of the shame and part of the silence is because in this society we are not encouraged to talk about our bodies. It's just not an open topic among women and your friends.'

It's really not. It amazed me that I could be a second-time mum and still so wide-eyed when it came to my postpartum recovery, or lack of it. Even more so when I came to realize how common these problems were. But Peace is right. It wasn't talked about. I had friends who'd had babies, friends who have seen me at my absolute worst, but we just didn't go there. During my first pregnancy I remember naively asking why I needed pads in my hospital bag. 'Don't worry about it,' they said. 'Just pack them.' There was nothing in the pregnancy books either. Not about prolapse or incontinence or healing after birth. I'd like to think that things are better now, but, bar a couple of exceptions (such as Emma Brockwell's recent triumph *Why Did No One Tell Me?*, which is essential reading and might have changed my entire pelvic floor journey had it been written a few years earlier), the pelvic floor remains barely a footnote. Weekly antenatal classes did little to prepare me either, apart from introducing me to a fabulous bunch of women who would all, eventually, be left wondering if they'd missed something among the knitted boobs and Marmite nappies. I will concede that pelvic floor squeezes were mentioned by the midwives at check-ups, but only ever in a slightly bashful tick-the-box kind of way. Not with any information behind it. Not in a way that made me consider what it was really all about.

So I can understand when people argue for pelvic floor health to be built into our preparation for birth, in every way and at every opportunity. But I don't actually think that's the answer, or at least not the whole answer. Hear me out. It's not because I agree with those who think pregnant women are too fragile to hear it – the idea that we shouldn't be trusted with information about our own health belongs in the dark ages. Neither do I agree with those who worry that it will push up C-section rates, because a) it's not necessarily true and b) it's not their decision to make. What I do think is that, by the time you're pregnant, it's too late. There's too much going on to start learning from scratch. There are too many other things on your mind. And once you've had a baby, it's definitely too late. Prevention doesn't work if it happens after the fact. And current thinking is that pelvic floor problems can, at least sometimes, be prevented.

Alongside a healthy lifestyle, the latest NICE guidelines recommend pelvic floor muscle training for *all* women throughout their lives to help prevent symptoms of pelvic floor dysfunction.[4] There are calls for more research on the long-term effectiveness of this, but just having that knowledge would be a start, because, again, imagine a world where Kegels weren't something to be whispered or embarrassed about. That in itself would be a game changer. So, to be clear, we should absolutely be talking about pelvic health during pregnancy and for the rest of our lives afterwards. But I'm convinced that we should also start by teaching it from a young age and in detail. It's a conclusion that Peace has also reached – when I asked her about it, she smiled and said she's hopeful that things will improve, as long as we don't keep the next generation in the dark: 'I feel for my sons because they're going to know way too much, but I think it's essential to educate our children not just about the basic things and the things that are expected of them, but the things that will happen, that nobody wants to talk about.'

When I was at high school in the nineties, the pelvic floor did not get a look in. I remember being taught the basics of reproduction, and how to avoid it (in an abstinence kind of a way). We learned to label the internal reproductive system – the vagina, uterus, fallopian tubes, cervix and ovaries – but not much else. Not the wider pelvic anatomy, nothing about the vulva, nothing about female desire and *obviously* nothing about pleasure. We weren't taught that the muscles of the pelvic floor play an important role in sexual function. We definitely weren't taught about the clitoris. Perhaps that's not surprising, seeing as, for centuries, it was ignored or misrepresented, barely even mentioned in the medical textbooks. It wasn't until 1998, which, for reference, was four years after the Spice Girls were formed, that the Australian urologist Professor Helen O'Connell led the first comprehensive anatomical study of its actual size and scope. She blew everyone's minds when she discovered that the clitoris was much bigger and more complex than anyone had previously thought, prompting a rewrite of anatomy books and helping to preserve sexual function during pelvic floor surgery.

So no, I didn't learn about female pleasure in school. As far as education went, the male orgasm was the ultimate goal, and only ever for the purpose of procreating. And I'm sure of this, because in a totally non-scientific survey of old school friends on WhatsApp, no one could recall learning anything else. 'Periods and not getting pregnant' was how one described it. 'I only recently learned the whole thing is the vulva,' said another. 'I thought it was all the vag.'

Twenty years later, when the pelvic health physiotherapist Tiffany Sequeira was at high school (and after the anatomy of the clitoris had been well established), I'm afraid to say not much had changed. When I spoke to her for the podcast, she told me, 'I went to an all-girls school until I was eighteen. I could do algebra. I could name all the parts of a plant. I could name all this random stuff, but I could not name you the anatomy of the vulva, the vagina. I could not label five things on a female pelvic anatomy. And I think, gosh, there is something that we're really doing wrong here.'

These days Tiffany is on a mission to educate. She told me that, when she realized how little pelvic health information was available, especially for young people, she set herself up as @gynaegirl on Instagram, putting out much-needed information about, as she put it, 'Sex, vulvas, willies, wee and lots more . . .' She said she was motivated by the questions she was getting from her friends in their twenties: 'I would think, "How do you not know these things? How bad that we were not taught the basics!" I think it's getting better, and I think especially the Gen Zers are more open to talking about sex and relationships, which is great, but what I like to focus on are the things we don't like to talk about with sex or pelvic health. Stuff that actually happens to a lot of us but nobody ever mentions.'

As well as getting the information out there in the first place, Tiffany is passionate about making pelvic health more inclusive, because how else will you make it relevant to everyone who needs it? She said when her mum was pregnant, as an Indian woman, there was nothing she could relate to, and when Tiffany started working as a physio she noticed how every diagram or illustration she saw was of a white model, with a flat tummy and perky boobs. 'Who are we kidding here?' she said. 'Have brown skin, have black skin, have stretch marks and pubes. We're not all bog standard.' Not one to sit around doing nothing, Tiffany convinced a graphics student to design some pelvic floor models of women with brown skin and started using them in clinic. 'It's crazy', she said, 'that I'm having to source someone to do that.'

A woman messaged me once to tell me that the podcast was her 'main source' of pelvic floor information. And, in the nicest possible way, she pointed out that that was 'ridiculous'. And she's quite right. Here was someone who'd been having problems since giving birth eighteen months earlier, problems which she described as 'terrifying at worst' and 'life-altering at best', and the podcast was the only place she could find the information she needed? I'm hugely proud of *Why Mums Don't Jump*, and trying to fill that void is one of the reasons it exists, but when you think about it, it *is* ridiculous that basic information is so hard to come by. Help and support should be freely available to everyone who needs it – we shouldn't have to rely on podcasts or scour internet forums or social media for it. Knowledge about our bodies, and what we go through as women and as mothers, should be baked in from an early age.

As I write, pelvic health is not specifically covered in the school curriculum for England. Then again, relationships and sex education only became compulsory in 2020 and remains controversial in some quarters. There are reasons to be optimistic though; there are signs that things are changing. The latest NICE guidelines now also recommend that, from the age of twelve, girls are taught in school about pelvic floor anatomy, pelvic floor muscle exercises and how to prevent pelvic floor dysfunction.[5] This is music to my ears, and I really hope it happens, because when researchers in the US gave a group of teenage girls one lesson a week for six weeks, they found that knowledge improved 'significantly'. The teens understood the possibilities of pelvic floor muscle training, they knew that leaking wasn't normal and they knew the right names for their own anatomy.[6]

The hope is that this kind of education will help to

prevent problems before they start, or at least help women to be aware of symptoms and what action they might take – to know what is normal and what should not be accepted. And, by the way, this doesn't mean we teach these things *only* to girls, because the last thing we need is more 'secret women's business'. It's for everyone. And at a minimum it's going to help with a baseline awareness, which is going to help to minimize the taboo. To me, it's a no-brainer. An *opportunity*.

'If you know the words and the parts of your pelvis,' explained Tiffany, 'your vagina, your vulva, your clitoris, then if you've got any issues, you're more able to explain what's going on. We all have a pelvis, we all have private parts. It's nothing new, it's nothing dirty, yet everyone shies away from talking about it. That's what I'm really trying to push as much as I can, and I hope that one day in future if I were to have children, they would be part of an era where they can talk about things openly and freely without any kind of judgement there.'

Sounds good, right?

Your Privates

- One in three women is unable to label the vulva on a diagram, often getting it mixed up with the vagina.[7]
- Fewer than half of those questioned for a 2021 study knew that a woman has three holes in her private parts.[8]
- NICE health guidance recommends that, from the age of twelve, girls are taught in school about pelvic floor anatomy, pelvic floor muscle exercises and how to prevent pelvic floor dysfunction.[9]
- It's vital that we have an understanding of our anatomy so that we can recognize when something isn't 'normal' and have the language to ask for help.

CHAPTER 4

SARA

(THE HEAD GAME)

I've been staring at a blinking cursor for far too long, typing sentences and then deleting them. Annoyingly, I find articulating my feelings around my pelvic floor problems almost as difficult as talking about my vagina. But the impact on your mental health is woven into the very fabric of this book. Because, obviously, no one is fine with their insides threatening to escape, or with leaking, or with living in pain. I've sometimes wondered if my issues are *more* of a head game than anything else. It's not that the physical symptoms aren't there, it's just that the emotional toll has sometimes been harder.

In the weeks and months after my son was born, I was a bit of a mess. I was. But isn't everyone? Even now it's hard to know how much of it was because of a ruined undercarriage and how much was down to the exhaustion and feeding traumas that so often come with new babies. It wasn't a crisis, we were surviving, but it worried the health visitor enough to prescribe a course of baby massage for me and my son, where everyone else seemed to be having an equally difficult time and which, I now know, has been shown to help with postpartum depression – a 'mad mums club' as one classmate jokingly described it. It did help. And, over time, things became more manageable.

My physiotherapy referral came through when my son was around a year old. Over a series of five sessions I developed what was deemed to be an acceptable level of pelvic floor strength and benefited from some much-appreciated emotional support. Then I was discharged. So I thought that was it, that I had reached the limit of my physical and mental recovery, and I tried to get on with finding my new normal. I was back at work by this point, and my husband and I were doing our best to contain and nurture a lumbering toddler and his three-year-old sister. Sensible levels of sleep were still a distant memory, but we were doing OK. The kids were wonderful and hilarious and in lots of ways everything was good, but my prolapse still bothered me. The bulge was still there, and it was on my mind a lot. Not every waking moment, but let's say . . . most of them.

For the next few years it was a limiter on life that made me think twice about almost everything I did: lifting a heavy bag, running for a bus, carrying an errant child down the road. I felt fragile and weak. I was grieving for the person I was and for the mum I believed I would never be. On some level I blamed myself: for not preparing well enough for birth, for not looking after myself afterwards, for taking my body for granted. I felt out of control and not in a wild-night-out kind of way, but just broken, decrepit. Even if you knew me, you wouldn't have known any of this. It's not like I was crying all the time or unable to function. At its worst, it was more of an absence of feeling, alongside total fatigue. I remember sitting in the parked car one day, looking at my seat belt and thinking that just the act of unbuckling it seemed like a lot of effort. We were on a family trip to a museum and I shuffled along the pavement behind everyone, trying to muster some enthusiasm. It wasn't particularly cold, but I was freezing. It was like all the colour had drained away. I had no energy, no interest, no words. The kids were zipping around the old planes and trains, pointing at the displays and having a lovely time. But I felt frail, disconnected from the world. And then I felt guilty because I should be more grateful for these beautiful, healthy children. I should be happy.

I'm sharing this not because I think that my story is special, but precisely because it isn't. I hear regularly from women who tell me that their problems have taken them to a dark place – that they've spiralled, and suffered alone because they've been unable to talk about any of it, sometimes even with those closest to them. Women who ran marathons and who now struggle to walk, who are dealing with 'feelings of shame, guilt, confusion and total isolation', questioning whether they should have done something differently, overwhelmed by what they feel they have lost. And shocked, so shocked, because no one warned them this could happen. So no, my story isn't special, and neither is it extreme. For many others, things are harder.

Research suggests that women with pelvic floor dysfunction are three times more likely to suffer from symptoms of depression than those without.[1] It's associated with a poorer quality of life and is linked to isolation and loneliness, which have *also* been shown to lead to depression and anxiety. It's pretty obvious when you think about it – if you're in pain, or discomfort, or there's a chance that you're going to wet yourself, or soil yourself, that's going to affect everything you do, from the school run to a night out, from a gym class to a business meeting. You'll worry about making things worse, about smelling, about being 'found out', so you'll have the strain of hiding it too. It will affect your self-esteem and body image, which in turn will affect relationships and intimacy.[2,3] And of course, it's embarrassing and shameful, which is magnified because it is so hard to talk about this most personal part of your body.

Don't forget that pelvic floor problems are more likely to happen if you've had a difficult vaginal delivery – maybe forceps, maybe a long labour or tearing – so there's a good chance that you're processing a tough or frightening birth at the same time.[4] The Birth Trauma Association estimates that around 30,000 women experience birth trauma every year in the UK, which can lead to symptoms of post-traumatic stress disorder (PTSD): flashbacks, anxiety or feeling constantly alert.[5] And that's all on top of the life-changing transition you're making into parenthood. There is layer upon layer of stress to wade through. Your vulnerability is off the scale.

Dr Rebecca Moore is a perinatal psychiatrist and co-founder of Make Birth Better, which campaigns to raise awareness of birth trauma. She specializes in caring for women with mental health issues, especially through

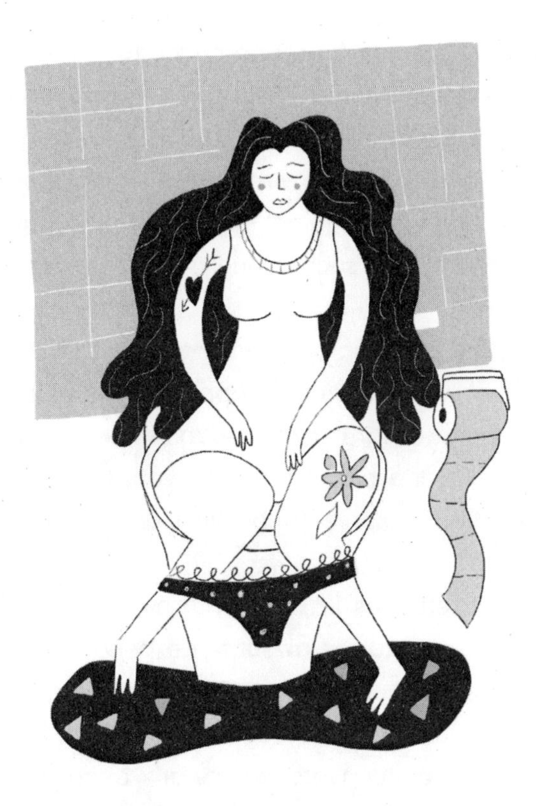

pregnancy and in the first year after childbirth. She was one of the first guests on the podcast and she has seen the profound impact these injuries have on women's lives:

> Most people that I sit with have got any one of a huge variety of mental health symptoms going on. Not necessarily a diagnosis, but they're struggling to make sense of what happened. They feel low. They feel anxious. They feel guilty. They feel angry. They feel distressed in lots of different ways. I think it's really often missed, and that we

> don't give women time and space to talk about how it feels to have these injuries . . . if you're a twenty-nine-year-old, thirty-nine-year-old, whatever-age-you-are woman, and suddenly you're left with a prolapse or incontinence and yet you're not expected to talk about that or voice that, it's just such a lonely, difficult place to be.

We really *don't* give women the space to talk about this. I don't know why. I think it's all wrapped up in the it's-normal-when-you-have-children attitude. You think everyone else is getting on with life and so should you. Maybe you don't realize that you deserve to be well or that you can ask for help.

Sara Duckett lives in Essex with her husband and two children. She wrote to me about her experience of incontinence and when I asked if she would let me share her story on the podcast, she agreed. We recorded remotely in early 2022 and I remember our conversation clearly, because she spoke with such openness and clarity of thought that she made me cry. You wouldn't have known this because I felt like a plonker afterwards and edited it out, but it left a mark.

Sara's problems began after her eldest son was born in 2016. She was induced, there were complications and she ended up with an episiotomy and forceps. It was rough. And the recovery afterwards? That was rough too: 'I was all over the place. I was having a lot of issues with leaking urine, not able to control anything, not able to exercise or walk because I would just basically wet myself. So I was having to wear the really big, thick pads to try to combat all of that.'

Sara was referred for physiotherapy, which began when her son was around six months old. She was given a programme of pelvic floor exercise, but after three months she was no better. She was told she would need an operation, but that if she wanted more children it would have to wait. And then she was discharged.

Like me, Sara thought that was it. That was as good as it was going to get. She was still leaking, and it was really starting to affect her self-esteem, but she struggled on for three years until she delivered her second son. It was a water birth, and she tells me it went amazingly well; it healed a lot of trauma. But her pelvic floor problems? They were worse. She was shocked to be told she had pelvic organ prolapse – something she had never heard of before. And now, not only was she not able to hold urine, but she wasn't able to hold a bowel movement either: 'When I started to leak poo as well, it was just . . . I didn't want to leave the house. I was very conscious all the time of, you know, the smell and stuff like that. And even though I never had an accident while I was out of the house, if I would walk particularly fast even, I would have some leakage when I got home. I was just so aware, hyperaware, of everything. It really took a massive toll on my mental health.'

Getting out of the house was one of the few things that kept me sane when I was looking after two small children. I remember breathing a sigh of relief every time we made it around the corner and over the road. We all did. However bad the night had been, however difficult the morning, we were out now, and the world was full of possibilities. During the Covid pandemic, new mums couldn't get out if they wanted to. For a long time, they couldn't see friends or family or compare notes at a baby group. There was precious little in the way of face-to-face support, on top of the worry of catching or transmitting Covid, and, unsurprisingly, levels of postpartum depression soared.[6] We just don't do well with social isolation, especially at such a difficult time in our lives, regardless of whether it's mandated by the government or self-imposed.

Sara told me she withdrew from friends. She didn't want to leave the safety of home because her incontinence had reached a point where it made it hard to do even the most basic of things. Going up and down stairs or just walking was a problem; a cough or a cold would be a disaster. She was carrying a lot: 'I would feel guilty for complaining about it, thinking, "Some people are so desperate to have children, some people can't have children, and I've got two beautiful children and yet I'm so unhappy." And I just felt like the odd one out all the time. My husband would be able to run about with them, and do different things, and pick them up in the park, and I just felt like I was on the sidelines, because I couldn't do any of that. It's really sad.'

Sara and I talked about how there's this societal expectation that parents, mums in particular, should sacrifice everything and anything for the sake of our children; that we should accept any level of suffering to keep them safe and well, and, of course, we would – 100 per cent, we would. But really, what our children need is for *us* to be well, or as well as we can be. Study after study has shown that maternal mental health is closely linked to the mental and physical health of our children. This is not to add to the guilt, but to say that it's not selfish to understand how important that is. We have to find a way to be thankful for our children *and* to know that we're important too. Easier said than done, I know.

'The more I was dealing with these issues,' Sara told me, 'the more my mental health was declining, and I didn't realize until I got to breaking point.' That breaking point came when Sara's second son was around six months old. He was in his highchair, eating lunch in the lounge when she urgently needed the loo. He had just started on solids and she was worried about him choking, so she felt she had no choice but to take him with her: 'I couldn't leave him eating because I knew it wasn't safe, so I had to drag him in the highchair to the downstairs toilet. And bless him, he was still eating his lunch while I was there on the toilet saying, "Sorry, sorry about this!" You know, they don't care, do they? But I was thinking I can't live my life like this. I can't carry on.'

It was affecting Sara's work too. She's a primary school teacher and felt uncomfortable and stressed about going in, wondering if she'd make it to the toilet in time. She couldn't just dash out of the classroom whenever she needed to, and she didn't feel like she could speak to her colleagues about it. On one occasion she had to leave work early because a cough was making her pelvic floor problems unmanageable. As if returning to work after having children wasn't hard enough.

In my job as a radio producer I would sometimes work on location to cover a news event. It was a privilege and I loved it, and in 2016 – when my son was around eighteen months old – I was sent to the Team GB 'Heroes' parade in Manchester, where thousands of people were lining the streets to celebrate Britain's success at the Rio Olympics and Paralympics. It was raining, of course it was, but there was an incredible atmosphere as the athletes drove through the city on open-top buses. I was due to be on one of the buses to produce a live broadcast, but the weather was causing technical havoc, so with just minutes to go it was suggested that I take the backup equipment – a hard-shell suitcase filled with maybe 15 kg of kit. My heart just stopped. I remember standing there like a rabbit caught in headlights, mentally speeding through my options. I didn't feel physically able to carry that kind of weight on and off buses and up and down streets for the next three hours, but I hadn't told anyone at work about my prolapse and no way could I reveal all now, not in the moment. So I mumbled something about a bad back and thankfully there wasn't any time for further explanation. As it happened, the skies cleared and the original gear held out, but making excuses for this unmentionable condition felt pathetic and shameful.

How *do* you tell your colleagues about your pelvic health issues? How do you tell your boss? It's a question that crops up a lot in this strange new world I have found myself in. I know of women who've made all kinds of excuses when they've been unable to cope with the physical strains of their jobs. And then the stress and guilt of lying about it makes it worse. Some have taken days off. Some have quit altogether. And it's so frustrating because maybe if these conditions weren't so stigmatized, honest conversations could happen and adjustments could be made.

I remember receiving a message from one listener who was off work, having called in sick that day. Let's call her Nina. She was really struggling with her prolapse symptoms – a painful dragging feeling, coupled with irritable bowel syndrome (IBS), in a job where she was on her feet all day, moving heavy equipment around, and where the only toilet was just one wall away from a row of desks, which made everything worse. 'I felt so awful mentally and physically,' she told me, 'I was broken.' She couldn't bring herself to explain any of it to her boss, so she said she had a headache, and then felt bad for lying, and not for the first time.

Nina later told me that a few days after sending that message, she felt able to go back to work and decided to speak to her boss about it. She mentioned 'IBS' and 'gynae stuff', said she was feeling really low and didn't like discussing it openly. Her boss was lovely. She told Nina to leave early or take a day off when she needed to, and not to worry as she knew how hard she worked. And she said she was sad that she'd been suffering at work. 'It made a big difference to me,' Nina told me. 'I was embarrassed, but I felt understood.' There's more good news too. With the support of a doctor and a physio, her IBS and prolapse symptoms have improved to the point where she's feeling much better. So much so that she gets up some mornings and dances . . . to drum and bass. What a way to start the day.

There's not a lot of research into the impact of pelvic floor problems in the workplace: how many women are taking sick days or have left their jobs altogether, how many are making excuses about bad backs or headaches because telling the truth is just too hard. But in 2005, researchers in the US surveyed more than 2000 women between eighteen and sixty years old and asked about their experience of urinary incontinence at work. They found that more than a third (37 per cent) had experienced unwanted urine loss in the previous month and that they were managing it by taking frequent bathroom breaks or wearing pads, but also by limiting fluid to keep an empty bladder, storing extra clothes or underwear at work, or by avoiding lifting, bending and reaching. For those with the more severe symptoms, it affected their concentration, physical activity and self-confidence.[7] This is no small impact. How do you do your job to the best of your ability when you're managing all of that? It can't be good for productivity, or for morale. It's not good for anybody. And with 15 million women in work in the UK alone, it's something we should be talking about.

It gives me hope to see workplaces starting to make changes when it comes to women's health – introducing menstrual leave, doing more to support employees through menopause and miscarriage – but we need to feel able to speak openly about *all* our health issues, and all managers need to be equipped to be able to listen and help, to make reasonable adaptations and to provide information about prevention and treatment. It was the podcast that finally forced me to tell colleagues about my problems. It wasn't easy; I found it embarrassing. But it was liberating too, because then it was out there, and I didn't have to carry it anymore.

On New Year's Eve in 2020, Sara was at a hospital appointment, having one of a series of tests to see which treatments she would need going forwards. She told me she joked with the nurse that this wasn't how she'd planned to bring in the new year, and then she broke down and told her how low she was feeling. It led to a call with her colorectal consultant, which led to a referral for counselling. And then slowly, over weeks and months, she started to feel better: 'It got me back on my feet again. It helped me to realize that it's a medical condition that I have, but it doesn't define who I am. I can still live my life and I can still go and do things, but I just have to make adaptations. And I think, now I've accepted what has happened to me, it's helped me to move forwards and to seek the right treatment, and not to settle for how things were.'

Sara told me that if she hadn't been offered therapy, she wouldn't have asked for it, because she just didn't know it was available. And that's why she wants to share her experience now, because getting the right support has made such a difference to her.

When I spoke to Dr Rebecca Moore she told me it's a process – that you have to be kind to yourself physically and mentally, but that small steps are still steps. And she says there are a hundred different ways to heal: 'It might be that you have therapy, so you have a space to process it and learn how to cope, and learn some practical skills around just managing those feelings day to day. It might be that you want to take medication. It might be about working with a physio as well. There might be dietary things you do. There might be supplements you take. There might be meditation. There's a whole host of different things and what I feel is that we need to offer women all of these choices.'

Sara realized she could ask for help and that she did have options – things she could try for her physical symptoms that might give her the life she wanted. She was offered a non-surgical treatment called Percutaneous Tibial Nerve Stimulation (PTNS), where a needle is inserted near the ankle and an electric current stimulates a nerve that controls the bladder and bowel. It's a sort of electro-acupuncture that's recommended by the NHS in some areas. Sara went for it, as well as getting a pessary, a plastic or silicone device that sits in your vagina to hold things in place (more on that later). She said the combination of the two has made a huge difference; she's back to exercising and doesn't need to wear a pad everyday: 'It's given me back the freedom to do normal things, just to have a normal life and do what I want with my children. It's like I've done a complete one-eighty from how I was, to how I am now. I just feel like I've got my life back.'

I asked Sara what advice she would have for her younger self. What she would say to herself when it all first happened, if she could go back in time and say it. 'That it's not your fault,' Sara said (and this is when we both choked up). 'I spent such a long time feeling like I was a failure; that I had failed at giving birth, I'd failed breastfeeding. And I was just so, so hard on myself. I felt like I wasn't worth anything. I felt broken, completely broken. So I think the main takeaway is to say that you are worth looking after. It is worth going to the doctors and pushing to get the right treatment. You are worthwhile and you deserve it.'

Mental Health

- Research suggests that women with pelvic floor dysfunction are three times more likely to suffer from symptoms of depression than those without.[8]
- Support is available. Speak to your health practitioner about a referral to mental health services. You can refer yourself directly to the NHS talking therapies service (IAPT).
- There are organizations that support women with birth injuries like Make Birth Better, the Birth Trauma Association and MASIC.
- Please tell someone how you're feeling and be kind to yourself. Small steps are still steps.

CHAPTER 5

CHANTELLE

(THE TABOO)

I am easily embarrassed and in my younger days I would blush a lot. I still do a bit. Sometimes for good reason, sometimes for absolutely none at all – sudden attention from a teacher, a compliment from a friend, a question from a colleague or an unexpected exchange with a passer-by. The heat just creeps up my face. There's nothing I can do about it. And there's always someone there to point it out, which makes it worse. So no, embarrassment is not my friend, and I have found my pelvic floor problems really embarrassing. I am obviously not alone in this, but, until recently, I never really stopped to question it. Why are we so ashamed of anything remotely relating to our genitalia? We weren't born feeling like this, and historically it hasn't always been this way.

Dr Catherine Blackledge is the author of *Raising the Skirt: The unsung power of the vagina* (originally published as *The Story of V*, because, she says, in 2003 the publishers couldn't cope with the word vagina). She has waded through ancient texts to explore historical attitudes towards female genitalia and, when I spoke to her for the podcast, she explained that there was a time when having a vagina was a source of power and pride, commanding respect and authority: 'One of the most amazing things I came across when writing the book was the raising the skirt stories. There are so many of them; crossing millennia, crossing cultures, in mythology, in art, in folklore, in history. They all talk about the incredible power of the vagina – that if a woman deliberately raises her skirt to reveal her vulva, she can cause an array of extraordinary things to happen.'

Dr Blackledge told me that, for centuries, different cultures around the world believed that the act of a woman exposing herself could prevent evil, calm the elements and frighten away attacking animals. It was thought that 'raising the skirt' could make the ground fertile, and act as a form of protest. It was even used as a military tactic, with groups of women displaying all and sundry to frighten away the enemy. The vulva was feared and revered and then . . . it wasn't. Dr Blackledge explained that bad science, western religion and the morals of the day had a major role to play in this: women came to be seen as a reproductive resource and the vagina as a 'passive vessel' – nothing more than a channel for sperm in one direction and babies in the other. Sex for anything other than procreation became 'sinful', so our genitals were systematically veiled or hidden beneath a fig leaf. Our bodies were objectified, and we were conditioned to feel embarrassed and sometimes disgusted by them. It was even built into the language – the word 'pudendum', an anatomical term for the vulva, has its roots in the Latin for 'shame'.[1]

You can start to see how we might have arrived at this point. We have been taught to cover up and censor ourselves in every way. Periods are dirty. Female sexual pleasure is taboo. We think our vulvas are the wrong shape because we don't see enough realistic images to know what 'normal' looks like. Perhaps that's why labiaplasty, a surgical procedure to reshape the lips of the vulva, is one of the fastest growing trends in plastic surgery worldwide.[2] We're sold sprays, wipes and douches because, it's claimed, we require special cleansing rituals. (We don't. The vagina is designed to keep itself clean with the help of natural discharge.[3]) And we think we're too hairy because, well, porn said so. If this is how society feels about a fully functioning, standard-issue vagina, imagine how it feels about one that exists in a world of damaged pelvic floors and fallen internal organs. Imagine how it feels if we then throw the uncontrollable leaking of private bodily fluids into the mix. All of this is such a taboo that it would be a miracle if we were not at least a little bit embarrassed.

But what are taboos, really? They are customs, invented by people, and then handed down from one generation to the next. Some of them make a lot of sense (murder, cannibalism – that sort of thing). But, as far as I can see, this one serves no useful purpose and, at its worst, prevents us from understanding our own bodies, stops us from seeking medical help and then leaves us feeling isolated and ashamed. So why don't we just change it? I know. I know it's not as simple as that. But we've started talking openly about loads of things that were once considered taboo – like mental health, like menopause, like periods, like infertility. Vagina-owners make up half the world's population. If we start speaking out, maybe we can reinvent that custom. Maybe we can change the narrative.

Chantelle Sandham is speaking out. She's been managing bowel incontinence since having her third child in 2017 and was the first person to discuss it with me on the podcast. I'll always be grateful to her for putting herself out there and for talking so openly about what is one of the most stigmatized conditions in healthcare. 'Obviously it's shameful,' she said. 'It's embarrassing, it's uncomfortable and it's a taboo subject, isn't it? It's just not socially acceptable to go and poo yourself anywhere. So you can't go about thinking, you know, it's my problem and I'm not bothered what people think. You just can't.'

I first came across Chantelle on Instagram, where she was sharing her experience of birth injury as @tears_from_tearing. She only lives a few miles away from me, so, despite the Covid pandemic, we were determined to meet in person. When we finally got to record, it was in a local park and seven degrees outside. We sat on a bench, the obligatory two metres apart, with a cold wind and some overly friendly dogs playing havoc with the microphones, but it was so nice to be able to speak to her in person. Chantelle is down-to-earth and funny with it, and we talked until our teeth started chattering.

Bowel incontinence (or faecal incontinence) is the inability to control bowel movements. Again, it's difficult to estimate how common it is because it depends on who you ask and how you define it, but studies suggest that it affects up to one in ten women after childbirth.[4] Numbers will be higher if you include those with difficulty holding wind, which may sound trivial but can be mortifying for those affected; or if you include those who only have infrequent episodes, which again, may sound bearable but it isn't, because how do you plan your life knowing you could have an accident at any time? Obviously it's shrouded in taboo, highlighted by the fact that if you survey women face to face, you'll get lower numbers than if you do it online or by post.[5] And it's under-reported: fewer than one in three see a doctor about it, either because they're embarrassed or because they think it's 'normal'.[6]

Chantelle had a difficult first labour, but when she had her second baby everything was fine, so she thought this third birth would be straightforward again. It wasn't. She ended up with a forceps delivery and a bad tear, and when she got home, things were tough. For the next few weeks she was in pain and having problems making it to the toilet. She was worried, but she thought maybe she was over-reacting: 'I knew I was in a lot of pain and thought something wasn't right, but everyone kept saying to me, "You've had a baby, you're going to be in pain" and I just thought that's the way it is. I was having some accidents while going to the toilet, but I thought that was because I was walking slowly. I never even thought about bowel problems from having a baby, ever.'

At her six-week check, Chantelle mentioned her concerns to the GP who examined her and referred her to a gynaecologist. She didn't know it at the time, but she had damage to the anal sphincter, the pudendal nerve (a major nerve in the pelvis) and the pelvic floor, as well as a rectocele (a prolapse involving the back wall of the vagina) – all of which are associated with bowel incontinence.

To look at Chantelle, you obviously wouldn't know any of this; she was thirty-two when we met – fresh-faced and full of smiles. But when I asked her how she manages day to day, she told me it changes 'absolutely everything in your life'. She said accidents can happen anywhere, at any time. That she gets up early every morning to try to empty her bowels or to do a home enema before the rest of the house wakes up. She takes medication and carries spare clothes everywhere. Nothing can be last minute or unplanned. At one point she wouldn't eat all day, to try to avoid having an issue at the office, and she told me she barely remembers the first year of her son's life. She thinks it's her brain blocking out the memory of a really stressful time:

> When everyone was going to playgroups or enjoying things with their babies, I didn't really get to do those things, but I don't really remember the things that I did do with him, even if it was just at home. I look back at pictures from the first year and I don't really remember "Oh an aunty got that jumper" or "I remember that day". I don't recall that, which is strange because I can remember it from my first baby ten years ago.

For a long time, Chantelle said, she didn't really talk to anyone about what was happening, not even to her partner. She said he knew things were difficult, but not the full extent of it. And she told me it took its toll on their relationship: 'We've been together for fourteen years, there's not much we get embarrassed about . . . but it impacts all of that. And then there's other tension, isn't there, and at one point he was probably wondering why I wasn't being intimate with him . . . so yeah, that's the impact at home.'

Navigating intimacy after having a baby is difficult at the best of times. Apart from feeling like you've been run over by a bus, you're now looking after a small person, and you're exhausted; both parents are. That's enough to strain any relationship. Add pelvic floor problems to the mix and it can feel virtually impossible. Maybe you have pain during sex or you're afraid it will make your problems worse; maybe you're worried about leaking, or it's had such a negative effect on your body image that you can't face close contact – all of that is going to kill the mood, to say the least. And what about if you go on to meet a new partner? How on earth do you approach all of that with them? When researchers in the US surveyed more than 300 women about this, they found that symptoms of pelvic floor dysfunction were 'significantly' associated with reduced arousal, painful sex and problems reaching orgasm.[7] It's an issue women quietly email me about: how can they feel good about themselves when they feel so broken? Where can they go for help? No one tells you how to manage it, and the shame associated with it is debilitating; a taboo within a taboo.

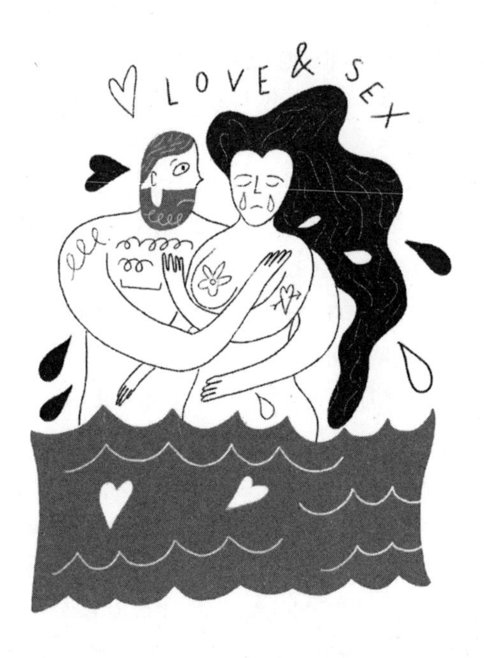

Jilly Bond is a pelvic health physiotherapist who treats women with intimacy problems after childbirth. When I spoke to her for the podcast she told me it can take years for women to seek help and that, when they finally reach her, it's often the first time they've felt able to discuss it: 'We ask about your bladder, about your bowel, about how everything is feeling in the vagina . . . and then we ask about intimacy. And they're not embarrassing questions, they're just "Are you achieving what you want to?" – because everyone has sex in a different way and it doesn't mean penetration, it can be lots of different things – but that tends to unlock a whole mass of problems that can occur, that people have never had the opportunity to talk about.'

Jilly said treating it is about taking a staged approach: addressing the physical symptoms, which can obviously be significant, but also the psychological side of things – fear, trauma, a sense of being broken. She said it might also mean working alongside psychosexual services – doctors, nurses and therapists who are trained in counselling around intimacy problems; a whole area of medicine that I had never heard of until we spoke. She said the hardest thing is asking for help in the first place, but, once you're there, there's always a way to improve things: 'All of these issues are so fixable and so remediable – I struggle to find in my mind anyone that we haven't been able to make progress with . . . It's like having a bad back, you know? We can get things moving.'

Over time, Chantelle opened up to her partner: she realized she needed to tell him more, she needed to ask for help. She was having treatment but her problems were no better. During the Covid pandemic they got worse and she had to give up work. She was waiting for surgery, but lockdown meant she didn't know when that would be: 'The not knowing has been the most difficult thing. Especially when it came to my son's birthday, because I was thinking, "It's been three years I've been like this" when really I should have been thinking, "I've done really well to get through the last three years."'

As we sat on the park bench, looking down across the playing fields, Chantelle told me she was trying to reprogram her thinking, to be more positive. She'd been having counselling, which had helped, but she said the biggest turning point for her had been finding support online, and realizing that she isn't the only person this has happened to:

> I saw a post from somebody that was about this, and they were pooing themselves . . . and I thought now there's two people in the world that poos themselves! So I messaged them, started a bit of a conversation and they said you should try this page and that page, and the next minute there were hundreds of women that were having the same issue. I was really sad that there were so many other people, but obviously . . . you're not alone are you?

The realization that you're not on your own is a game changer. The relief is enormous. And meeting other women is what inspired Chantelle to want to speak out. After that, she said she wasn't embarrassed to talk about it anymore. She started her Instagram account and agreed to speak on podcasts like mine; she got involved with the charity MASIC; and she set up a WhatsApp group. 'We're called the Fairy Bum Mothers,' she told me with a grin, 'and we just talk about poo every day.' She said it helped a lot.

When my son was three, I reached a turning point of my own. It happened during a trip to the Trafford Centre, of all places – a vast, indoor shopping mall that brings a touch of Vegas to the outskirts of Manchester. It's hard to miss with its glass domes, Grecian columns and semi-naked statues, but, as every local mum will tell you, its star attraction (if you're under the age of six) is the dolphin fountain in the middle. I've spent many a rainy afternoon with two small children throwing pennies into that fountain and it's where a chance encounter helped me to start talking.

It was May 2018. I was there, trying to stop the kids from falling into the water, and I ended up chatting to another mum. She was on her way to a nearby trampoline park, so you can imagine how that conversation went and, before I knew it, we had both declared our prolapses. It might sound innocuous, this small act of sharing, but I don't think I'd spoken so openly about it before then and it helped me to believe that this was a discussion it was possible to have. She recommended a local pelvic health physio and passed me the details, which prompted me to think again about what I could do to improve my situation. Maybe I hadn't reached the end of my recovery journey after all. Maybe we *could* talk about it. I *wanted* to talk about it. I wanted to vent. I wanted to connect with other women in the same boat. Four months later I set myself up on Instagram as @whymumsdontjump.

Someone asked me recently where the name came from, and I wish there was an inspiring and elaborate story behind its origin, but in truth it just popped into my head – an accidental pun on the 1992 film, *White Men Can't Jump*. You know the one, where Wesley Snipes and Woody Harrelson are basketball hustlers? There are parts of my subconscious that will forever be stuck in the early nineties. Anyway, it was catchy and it said everything it needed to. It was meant to be. As for why I chose an image-based social media platform to share my broken bits with the world... I have no idea. Back then, the 'gram was all sunsets, holiday snaps and food styled to perfection, definitely not this. I posted an illustration of my prolapse, anonymously, using an app called POP-Q, which converts the measurements from a pelvic floor exam into a computerized cross section of the real thing. It's a diagram – there's nothing X-rated about it – yet still I felt the need to add a black and white filter to make it more palatable:

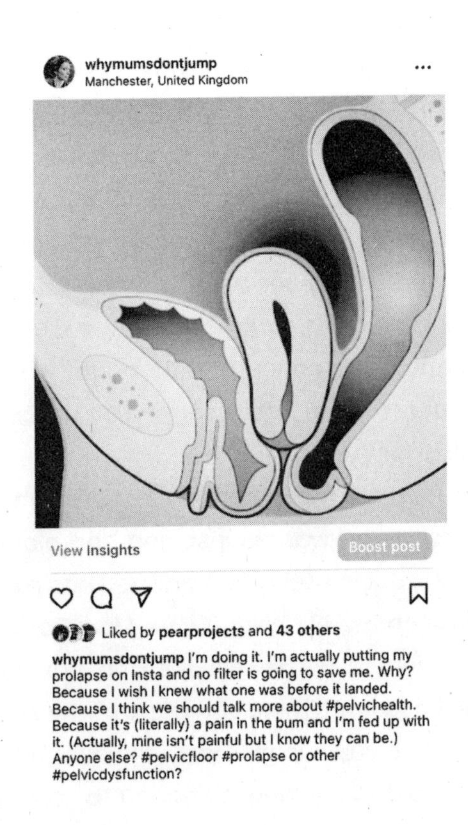

If I was worried that people would be disgusted or outraged, they weren't. They were kind and supportive, relieved to hear someone else talking about it. And they were sharing their own stories of prolapse, of difficult births and bladder issues. At the time, the only person I told in *real* life was my husband, Paul. 'Whatever you need to do,' was his response. The perfect response. Quiet reassurance has always been his superpower.

So there I was, happily posting away, anonymously, interacting with other mums, with physios and postnatal trainers – safe in the knowledge that nobody knew who I was. Then someone I knew started following the account and the world stopped spinning for a moment, because did they know it was me? *How* did they know? I later discovered that they didn't. I can only assume it was something to do with the infamous 'algorithm', but it was a shock, to say the least.

Not long after, I realized that if this was going to be a real conversation then I couldn't hide. So I had a stiff drink and put my name on my grid . . . and my face. 'I'm crap at selfies,' the caption read, 'and if you'd told me a year ago I'd be sharing this stuff on social media I would have said you needed to give your head a wobble. But here I am. #OutOfMyComfortZone.' I shed a little tear when those comments started rolling in. At that moment, some of the shame I was carrying started to lift. This is how it is with taboos – when you start talking, you break the spell. Besides, I'm not sure the algorithm would have let me get away with staying anonymous for much longer, because, by then, *four* people I knew were following the account without realizing it was mine. I'm relieved to say that when I put my name on it, they quickly got over their surprise and were full of encouragement and positivity. One had a prolapse herself, something that she too had been struggling with and something that we hadn't talked about until then – it was comforting to see a familiar face. Then I was out there. And I wouldn't have known how to delete it all, even if I'd wanted to.

More than a year after our chilly meeting in the park, I managed to catch up with Chantelle, and she told me that when surgery got up and running again after the initial Covid response, she was put back on the waiting list. Hospitals were reviewing patients and, understandably, prioritizing those who were felt to be in most urgent need. But Chantelle was given a priority level 4, the lowest category, which meant the operation could be delayed for three months or for much longer. It was devastating news. 'I wrote to the surgeon and said, "I know I'm not dying from this, but I feel like my life is just withering away",' she told me. 'I was so down that I felt like I was dying inside.' Chantelle knew it sounded dramatic, but it was how she felt. By that point, every day was a struggle. Chantelle's case went before a panel and, to her great relief, she was bumped up the list. She finally got her operation in May 2021, but she questions why she had to reach rock bottom to be seen as a priority and to access the treatment that she so badly needed.

Recovery isn't linear, things aren't perfect, but the surgery has made a huge difference to Chantelle's life. She's been able to do things again that most of us take for granted, like travelling on a train to meet a fellow Fairy Bum Mother, a long journey that she couldn't have risked before. She and her partner got married and she began training as a midwife. She knows the surgery has a lifespan, but by then her children will be older, and who knows what other treatments are coming down the line. In the meantime, she's on a mission, not to normalize bowel incontinence, but to show others that they're not alone, that there's someone else going through it and that they can talk about it, if they want to: 'I want to show that we're out there, that there's somebody else. And even if one person feels a bit better about it, then I feel like the mission's accomplished.'

Bowel Incontinence

- Bowel incontinence (also known as faecal incontinence) is the inability to control bowel movements and is estimated to affect up to one in ten women after childbirth.[8]
- Numbers will be higher if you include those with difficulty holding wind, which may sound trivial but can be mortifying. (The inability to control bowel movements *or* wind is known as anal incontinence.)
- Severe tears which damage the anal sphincter (OASI) are a common cause.[9]

- Treatments are available, so if you experience symptoms, please do not put up with them. Ask a GP or another healthcare professional for help.
- Remember, you are not alone.

CHAPTER 6

SOPHIE

(FINDING FITNESS)

It's October 2019 and I'm quietly bawling my eyes out in a consultation room, choked up unexpectedly during a physio appointment. It's hard to get the words out, but I manage it eventually: 'Happy tears . . . happy tears.' I've just been told it's not completely out there to think I could run again.

It sounds dramatic, I know, but I honestly thought that door had been closed to me for good. I had accepted that I would never again move faster than a brisk walk. That if I did, I was inviting my pelvic floor problems to get worse. And if that happened, I would never forgive myself. So it just wasn't worth the risk.

It's a weird one too, because I've never been a massive runner. As a teenager I used to run up hills with my dad; as an adult I ran occasionally – it's not like it was a great passion of mine. But the idea that I would never do it again really bothered me. I would watch other women jogging past, and resent the fact that I couldn't. I think it was a touchstone for all the other things I felt unable to do.

I mentioned it earlier, The Fear – how, so often, the advice is not to run or jump or lift anything heavy, but how you're not told what that looks like in real life or what you can do instead; how that becomes a barrier for every action you take. It's ageing, and paralysing: lose weight but avoid high-impact, no sit-ups, no aerobics, only lift your kids if you have to, no prolonged standing. We think we're protecting women, but in truth we're terrifying them into avoiding not only exercise, but any kind of movement at all. It's hard to explain how demoralizing it is to stop yourself every time you come close to the action – sitting on the sidelines, looking to someone else every time the kids want you to join in. We know that exercise brings with it huge benefits for physical and mental health, but there's a knowledge gap when it comes to its relationship with the pelvic floor and that's not OK.[1] It makes me so cross that we have been writing off a whole section of society in this way, seemingly without a second thought about the long-term consequences.

While we're at it, why, in 2022, are we still using housework as a reference point for physical activity? Bending to do the laundry? Standing to do the washing up? I just read a patient information leaflet that gives 'two hours of ironing' as an example of what not to do, as if there's no other conceivable reason for a woman to be on her feet. But I digress . . .

Running *is* a great passion for Sophie Power. She's an ultrarunner who takes on the longest and hardest races she can find, usually over 100 miles at a time. Yes, 100 miles. So when she was casually told, on the day after her first son was born, that she might not be able to run again, it was a devastating blow: 'It was the worst possible thing to say to someone who's a new mum for the first time and incredibly vulnerable. It was just, "You may never run again."'

When I spoke to Sophie for the podcast she told me that she had only found out what a pelvic floor *was* a few hours earlier, after she had given birth, and when she 'basically just peed myself everywhere'. She'd had an episiotomy and a ventouse delivery and it had taken its toll, but she was shocked to find herself leaking urine: 'I can't believe I got through my entire pregnancy without someone telling me that this could happen. And I know they kind of talked about it in pregnancy yoga, the squeeze and things, but no one explained that you could end up leaking.'

After the birth, Sophie spent three months without taking a running step. This, for her, was unheard of, and she struggled. It was 2014 and, if there was any help available, she couldn't find it. If she wanted to get back to where she was, she was on her own.

'Those three months were very, very difficult and I'm fairly sure that if I had seen someone I would have been diagnosed with postnatal depression . . . I vowed from there that I need to be on top of this. I need to know what's happening; I need to take control of my body; I need to research everything. And for all my friends who are going to have babies, I need to tell them what could happen, so that they don't have to go through what I did.'

Everything Sophie read seemed to say don't do anything, but she started really listening to her body and taking things step by step. She was making it up as she went along, but she was slowly getting fit again. She'd been doing strength training throughout her pregnancy, which she said really helped, and, bit by bit, her pelvic floor issues improved. By the time her son was six months old, she had done her first fifty-mile run.

Sophie was on my radar for a long time before I started the podcast. She had her second baby in 2018 and completed the 106-mile Ultra-Trail du Mont-Blanc when he was just three months old. Sixteen hours into a forty-three-hour mountain race, she stopped at a rest station and was photographed breastfeeding her son and pumping at the same time. She didn't think twice about it – he had to be fed and she needed to express – but the picture went viral around the world. It sparked a debate about motherhood and the unspoken pressure on mums to be 100 per cent focused on the new baby, rather than on their own physical and mental health. It became about women getting back to themselves after childbirth, still feeling able to have goals and, importantly, being supported to get there. As Sophie put it: 'That we still matter, separate to our children. We don't just become "Mother".'

I was in awe when I saw that photo and, I won't lie, a bit envious. Not because I wanted to run up mountains, but because I felt that it wasn't as simple as that for me. I didn't know then that it hadn't been simple for Sophie either. The news reports at the time didn't mention pelvic floors and I worried for any mum who might feel like they too had to get back to peak fitness within weeks of having a baby. This was back when I felt that exercise was the enemy, when movement was dangerous. Now, I see it through different eyes. I see a picture of hope, of choice and of empowerment. Just out of shot, Sophie said her husband was trying to get her to eat a sandwich, while her friend was busily changing the batteries of her head torch and restocking her snack supply. It's about having dreams, whatever they might be, and being helped to achieve them:

> The picture meant so much to so many people and I guess it's given me this platform to help other mums follow their goals and stay healthy and advocate for themselves . . . making sure we get the right support to get us to where we *want* to be, not just able to walk down the road leak-free, pain-free.

I often hear from women who have been told, at one stage or another, that not being able to do the activity they love is 'no big deal'. But really, who gets to decide that? Yes, we want to be able to do the bare minimum – to function and to walk down the road leak-free, pain-free – but we should be able to reach for far more than that. We just need the knowledge and expertise to get us there.

When I recorded with Sophie, four years later, in 2022, she was seemingly full of energy, despite being up half the night with her kids, and despite a punishing training schedule for an ultramarathon qualifier where she would have to run around the same 400-metre track for 24 hours. 'It sounds bonkers,' she said, 'but it's really quite nice to have twenty-four hours where you don't have to think about anyone else.' I can almost see the attraction. Almost.

Sophie told me the photo had shown the world what was possible in terms of postpartum recovery, but she wanted to tell women *how* they could do it. So during her third pregnancy, she agreed to let a local photographer document her experience in a short film.[2] She didn't know what would happen – every pregnancy is different, every recovery is different – but she felt that if seeing her journey in all its honesty could help one woman, then it was something worth doing. It's how, six weeks after her third child, her daughter, was born, she came to find out she had a prolapse . . . on camera: 'I'd heard the word prolapse before but only in the context of "old women". I didn't think that was something that could happen or was common . . . it was a massive shock. And your mind goes straight to "Can I run again? What does this mean?"'

If you watch the film, you'll hear Sophie gasp when she's told she has a prolapse. It really stuck with me and I was trying to work out why. I think that, once again, it comes down to that sense that you're not the only one this has happened to. Knowing that someone else has experienced it all in a similar way and gone through some of the same emotions makes you feel seen, less alone, less of a disaster somehow. It's validating, and powerful.

This time, Sophie had the support she needed. After the photo went viral, she'd been invited to speak about her postpartum recovery at an exercise medicine conference – largely because there's so little research about how to do it – and that's where she met the pelvic health physiotherapist Emma Brockwell, who supported her throughout her third pregnancy. Emma was the one who delivered the bad news; fortunately, she had also just co-written the first ever UK guidelines on returning to running after childbirth.[3] No one was better placed to help Sophie get back to where she wanted to be.

I might have fangirled Emma a bit when I spoke to her for the podcast. She is a physio with first-hand experience of prolapse after childbirth, but she is also a runner and a huge advocate of exercise throughout pregnancy and beyond. 'You need to move, you *can* move, you possibly just need a little bit of guidance as to how to start, and how to make it work for you.' Having spent years avoiding all the things I thought I was supposed to avoid, here was someone saying it was possible to break a sweat without making things worse. Here was a reason to be hopeful. Emma told me that, up to now, there's been a conservative approach to movement when it comes to pelvic floor dysfunction, mainly because of a lack of research. We don't know, so probably don't do it. But things are changing: 'We've found that by holding women back, it's not changing symptoms. It's not necessarily making them any worse, it's definitely not making them any better. But we've got to a point now where we feel we can challenge the pelvic floor and its surrounding tissue . . . and we're learning and finding that, actually, women are reporting improvement, from a symptomatic point of view.'

Research around this is starting to emerge, but there's a long way to go. When the latest NICE guidelines were released, it felt to me like there was a small but welcome change in tone. Rather than 'don't do anything ever', it suggests that physical activity, alongside pelvic floor muscle training, may help with symptoms of pelvic floor dysfunction. Based on the studies available, it concludes that yoga and Pilates, when supervised, probably don't do any harm, and they might actually help.[4] So there's that. And then there's a big question mark over pretty much everything else, along with a call for more research so that the advice we give to women can be based on actual evidence. It doesn't seem like a lot to ask, especially when physical inactivity is such a big public health concern; when around the world we know that women are less active than men, and when the World Health Organization says that one in three of us are not doing enough physical activity to stay healthy.[5] Not when there's evidence that a mother's activity levels are directly linked to her children's.[6] It shouldn't be left to us to figure this stuff out by ourselves.

It took me four years to figure out my route back to fitness. I hadn't stopped moving completely in that time – I was cycling a short distance to work and I went to a weekly Pilates class for a while – but it felt risky, like I might be doing more harm than good. Planks and sit-ups were supposed to be bad, weren't they? Or were they? Nobody seemed to know for sure. And the internet turned up such contradictory advice that I didn't trust any of it. I tried a spin class too, but lost confidence when the instructor said she'd never heard of prolapse. She's not alone. Some fitness professionals *do* train in pre- and postpartum exercise and will have a level of knowledge about pelvic floor dysfunction, but others don't. A woman messaged me to say how shocked she was to find she had a prolapse after her daughter was born. 'I had no idea it could happen,' she said, 'which is extra scary since I'm a personal trainer and used to train mums.'

So I still held back on every urge to throw my kids around, dance with abandon or dig the garden. That was how it was, until that trip to the Trafford Centre. The physio I saw afterwards helped me to strip it back, to think about starting again and rebuilding my core which, I know now, is not just your abs but also your glutes, your hips, your lower back – pretty much all the muscles between your bra band and your bum, with your pelvic floor at the bottom. I learned that this is important, because all of these muscles work together, so you need them all to be in good shape, especially if a bunch of them are misfiring.

In January 2019, I tentatively signed up for an exercise programme with a focus on pelvic floor and core training – Holistic Core Restore. I was fortunate enough to be able to see a private trainer once a week and we got to work. It started gently with a lot of breath work, pelvic floor exercise and stretching, slowly progressing to squats and lunges, pulling, pushing and bending. I was following the programme, exercising to videos four times a week and I could feel the progression. My heart rate was up for the first time in years and, *crucially*, I felt safe doing it. This was progress for sure.

After around nine months I started working with a local yoga and Pilates teacher. You won't be surprised to hear that I got a bit emotional at my first session with Sadhana – I still felt vulnerable and here was someone who really wanted to help. She sat me down; she listened; she made really great ginger tea. And then she pushed me. I was lifting weights, even doing handstands against the wall, and I was getting stronger, more confident. It felt like I was putting myself back together, piece by piece. Maybe I could run after all. And if I could do that, then what else could I do? Maybe I could ditch The Fear for good?

That's how I came to be crying happy tears at a physio appointment and, after a bit more glute work, was given the green light to try running. There's a video of me getting ready for my first training session of 'Couch to 5K', a running plan for absolute beginners. You do sixty seconds of walking followed by ninety seconds of running for a total of twenty minutes. It's hardly extreme, but I was really nervous. It was a Saturday morning and I was doing an excellent job of procrastinating – watering a plant here, folding some laundry there, scrolling, pacing, doing anything to avoid putting my trainers on, because my head was telling me that my insides would fall out. Spoiler alert: they didn't. I eventually made it out of the door and into the autumn rain and it was completely exhilarating. I loved it. A few weeks in, my wonderful physio, Katie, came with me on a training run, which gave me even more confidence, and over six months I progressed to running

5 km around the local park, two or three times a week. My symptoms are no worse; sometimes I even think they're better for it. And it's made a huge difference to how I feel about my prolapse. I'm not as broken as I thought I was.

There is another, significant, side to this. For some, it's not The Fear, but the symptoms themselves that get in the way of exercise. If you leak when you run or you can't control your bowel movements, if you have heaviness in your vagina or pelvic pain, then that's obviously not a comfortable place to be, and it's common too – there is a reason for all those trampoline jokes. In 2018, researchers in Australia surveyed more than 4500 women with prolapse or incontinence, and asked about their physical activity. They were aged between eighteen and sixty-five. Some had children, others didn't. One in three said their symptoms were a 'substantial barrier' to exercise, that they stopped exercising as often, or stopped exercising altogether.[7]

When I asked Emma Brockwell about it, she told me that symptoms while you're exercising are a sign that your body isn't coping with the exertion you're putting it through, so you shouldn't just ignore it or whack on a pad. You do need to seek professional help. But it doesn't mean that fitness is finished. It might just mean paring things back, at least for a while: 'I don't necessarily think high-impact is for everyone. I need to be clear with that. But for most women, so long as we're being specific, and retesting and re-evaluating, we can formulate a programme that helps get you back to the exercise that suits you and that you like.'

For Sophie, recovery felt slow, and a torn hamstring didn't help. She missed the escapism, missed the adventure of running, but she also knew that if she rushed it, she could be risking everything, that things could get worse. So she took things step by step and, under the watchful eye of Emma and her running coach, her symptoms improved. She was fitted for a cube-shaped pessary (more on that later), which she nicknamed Poppy (because why not?) and, at nine weeks, she was able to start running again. Uphill to start with, then onto flatter surfaces, then trails, then downhill, and then racing.

It hasn't all been plain sailing. Sophie told me that when she got back to real strength, she got a bit complacent. She wasn't leaking anymore. She thought she was fine. So she stopped doing her pelvic floor exercises. And at her next check-up, two months later, Emma noticed a lack of strength. 'She gave me a big warning,' Sophie told me, 'and said it had gone down to a point that if I kept not doing them, the muscles wouldn't be strong enough to hold the pessary, and my mind was like "No pessary, no run. Right, OK. I'd better do them again." It was a big wake-up call that we're postpartum for life.'

I confess that my fitness has gone to pot lately. Life got a bit hectic, self-care went to the bottom of the pile and my training took a hit. I do some sporadic Kegels and I have managed to hang on to a weekly jog, but not much more, and I'm feeling it. It's different this time though. Because I know now that I can get it back and that I will. That the door isn't closed. The Fear hasn't left me completely – sometimes the doubt creeps back in. Like when I took the children bouldering a while back and got really confused about whether it would be wise to join in. But these days it doesn't restrict me in the same way, because I know more about what my body can and can't do. I know that it's about taking things one step at a time, and I know that I have people around me who can offer guidance and support, people who know way more about it than I do, who can set me back on track.

Pelvic Health Physiotherapy

- A pelvic health physiotherapist (or women's health physiotherapist) is a physiotherapist who is specially trained in the rehabilitation of the pelvic floor.
- They can assess and treat a wide range of pelvic floor problems and can help you safely return to exercise or activity.
- In the UK you can ask your GP to refer you, or in some areas you can self-refer. You can also pay to see a pelvic health physiotherapist privately.
- Symptoms while you're exercising are a sign that your body isn't coping with the exertion you're putting it through, so don't ignore them. Seek help.

CHAPTER 7

RACHEL

(YOU DON'T JUST PUT UP WITH IT)

I don't remember exactly when I decided to make a podcast about pelvic floor problems. There was no light-bulb moment. It was more of a dawning realization. I was getting all these messages from women who, just like me, were quietly struggling with these life-changing issues, and a thought became an idea and then something that I absolutely, without question, had to do. I'm rarely certain about anything, but I was certain about this. If we wanted to end the stigma, then we needed to share stories and accurate information, we needed to talk more openly, we needed to shout a bit louder.

I spent months thinking about it; taking advice from a few trusted colleagues, plotting out episodes, discreetly approaching potential guests. Then I went to a podcast festival to pick up some tips, which is when it all got a bit real because, on the way in, you had to write the title of your podcast on your name badge. I panicked briefly. Up to that point, barely anyone knew what I was planning, and here was a room full of people I'd never met, ready to network, ready to chat. But then there was a queue forming behind me, so I picked up a black marker pen and scrawled 'Why

Mums Don't Jump' across the label in capital letters. That was it. The more people I told, the easier it was to explain. They were kind, and if they were shocked, they hid it well.

I started recording, but, even then, I couldn't quite bring myself to launch. What would my family think? My colleagues? My friends? When I tell you what persuaded me in the end, you'll laugh. You know those motivational quotes you see when you're scrolling? 'Cake is the answer, no matter the question'; 'Create your own sunshine'; 'Do more of what makes you happy' – they're really not my thing, but then again maybe they are, because I was scrolling one day and I found the nudge I needed: 'It's better to create something that others criticize than to create nothing and criticize others.' Cheesy, I know. I was thinking it was someone like Tennyson, or Gandhi maybe, but it looks like it was the British comedian Ricky Gervais, in a Tweet from 2014.[1] Still, there you have it. It was April 2020, one month into the UK's first Covid lockdown and something about that quote, or the upended world, or the weather that day, made me set a date.

By this point, the number of people who knew about my plans was growing and I wanted to give my parents the heads-up before someone else did, but if I tell you that I grew up in a household where fart jokes were frowned upon, you'll understand that I had no idea where to start with this. They knew about my pelvic floor problems and were lovely about it, but how would they feel about me sharing them with the world in a podcast? How would *I* feel about them hearing it?

And yes, I am an overthinker, but I do think that these things are worth considering. We're not all ready to go full-on loudhailer about this. And although my current approach is to blurt out all the facts and pretend it's all as normal as discussing the weather, it isn't, not yet. We're all at a different level with it and will be for a while. And I think we can and should be sensitive to that. Anyway, lockdown saved me from a face-to-face conversation, and I emailed to let them know what was happening. Some would call it a cop-out. I would call it saving our blushes. 'Good luck,' was their reassuring response, 'where do we listen?'

So I pushed the button and scheduled the podcast to launch at 2 a.m. on a Monday morning. And by the time my alarm went off, I could see that dozens of people had already heard it. I spent the early morning stumbling around the house, sick with nerves. My heart was racing, my mind was too. I thought I might have inadvertently reduced myself to a broken vagina and there would be no going back, but I needn't have worried. Within hours, my DMs were flooded with heartfelt messages from women who told me it was the first time they'd heard someone say these things out loud; how they too were grieving for their old selves; how they had cried (and laughed) along with me, in supermarkets, on dog walks and in cars. They told me that hearing the podcast made them feel less alone, 'almost normal' again. They were sharing it with their partners and finding hints of hope. They asked me to 'please keep it up'. To say I was relieved would be an understatement.

A few weeks later I was amazed to find that at around the same time as I was pouring my heart out in that first episode, the journalist Rachel Horne was sharing her incontinence story with more than a million listeners on Virgin Radio. While I was hiding away and worrying in a makeshift bedroom studio, here was someone in the public eye chatting live on air about vagina weights (yes, that's a thing) while people ate their cornflakes. It was a real fist pump moment. I emailed her straight away. Rachel is the news presenter on *The Chris Evans Breakfast Show*. She grew up in Northern Ireland and spent a good chunk of her career at the BBC – presenting the children's news programme *Newsround* and then business bulletins on the BBC News Channel. She's witty, funny, articulate and a bundle of energy, despite getting up at an ungodly hour every day – one of those people who make you wonder how they fit it all in. When my email landed in her inbox, we were mid-pandemic and Rachel was broadcasting from her front room. She was elbow-deep in homeschooling three children and was too busy to think about recording just then but, as soon as things eased up, she got in touch to say she could do it.

For Rachel, it was an unexpected invitation to run the London Marathon that forced her to confront her pelvic floor problems. At the time, she wasn't a runner, for the simple fact that when she ran, she leaked. But her on-air colleagues, Chris Evans and Vassos Alexander, were very into running. They still are. They run marathons, they organize running festivals and they write running books. Vassos was writing a book about marathon training. Would Rachel be a case study?

> You know when your tummy drops? And I thought no, no, no, it's not me. And then I thought, I'm turning 40 and it's the London Marathon . . . what's stopping me? Well, what's stopping me is my pelvic floor. And actually, if I'm going to sort it, this is the perfect time to do it.

It was game on. Eight years after her first child was born, Rachel signed up to run 26.2 miles in one of the world's most famous marathons and to face down her incontinence. And when Chris asked her on air how training was going, she was ready to share. She took a moment, swallowed, and launched into it. It won't surprise you to hear that she was then inundated with messages from women thanking her for doing it. Me included.

Rachel had three vaginal births in three years; three 'savage' births, as she puts it. The first involved forceps and ventouse, and she tore badly on each occasion. She'd been through the childbirth wringer and then she did what so many of us do, she put herself to the back of the queue and got on with the not-so-easy task of looking after her three young children. There were still some problems, but hey that's normal when you've had kids, isn't it? (It isn't.)

> I was aware there were some issues, but it was nothing that was preventing me from doing what I felt I needed to

> do, which was keeping these three children alive. They become your priority and you fall down the list. So long as you're cleaned and clothed, nothing else is a priority.

Rachel told me that it was three years later when she realized she needed help. She was in her mid-thirties and wearing an incontinence pad most days. 'A bit of an issue' is how she described it when she finally went to see her GP and was put on the waiting list for physio. She started doing pelvic floor exercises and there was some improvement. So when the referral came through, Rachel decided that she was 'fine' and put it all back on the backburner. 'I think women can be very guilty of not putting our hands up and saying, actually, I need to be sorted, I need to come first and I need to be fixed. I was just like, "Look, there's been some improvement, I'll just keep doing the exercises. It's fine."'

It wasn't fine though. While we were on our video call, Rachel replayed a really difficult memory. It was emotional and it caught us both off guard. She told me how she was due to watch her son in a school concert. He'd been learning to play the saxophone for a couple of years, and she was determined not to miss the performance. Rachel was presenting TV bulletins at the time and had strategized her journey home down to the last detail. She came off air and rushed straight from the London studio onto the Tube in a full face of make-up. She made her train, got to the station, jumped in her car and drove to the school. She was getting texts from other mums telling her that she hadn't missed him, not yet. But she had to park quite far away from the school. So she got out of the car, and she ran. And as she ran, she leaked. And there was nothing she could do about it.

> I ran into the hall. I got in at the back just before he went up. And I saw him. And I was so proud of him. But I had to hold my bag in front of me. I was wearing a blue dress and it looked like someone had just thrown a pint of water at me.

It was visibly painful for Rachel to remember all of this. Through tears she told me that was when she decided she needed to wear a pad every day. It was another two years before the marathon challenge made her think again.

As we chatted, Rachel sneezed and simultaneously crossed her legs. We laughed about it. Of course we did. Sometimes you have to laugh, or you'd cry. But this is no joke. The adult incontinence market knows it's a serious business. Globally, it was valued at more than US$10 billion in 2020, with sales projected to rise over the coming years as the population ages.[2] On an individual level, it's estimated that if you're using pads every day, you could be spending up to £70 a month, more if you're using them at night as well.[3] And then there's the environmental cost of plastic waste from disposables. For many, these are truly invaluable products which can make life liveable; they are part of the solution as far as management is concerned. But they are also often criticized for masking and trivializing the problem – and of contributing to the 'normalization' of incontinence.

In the UK in 2019, there was an outcry over an advert for the disposable incontinence underwear, Tena Silhouette. You might remember it – where a new mum pulls on her jeans and says, 'A little bit of wee is not going to stop me being me.' The Royal College of Nursing complained to the Advertising Standards Authority saying it wrongly implied that bladder problems were inevitable after childbirth, and that protective underwear was the only solution.[4] The complaint was not upheld and Tena denied any wrongdoing, but, following the backlash, agreed to amend its adverts to encourage women with 'regular urine leakage' to seek healthcare advice.[5] A couple of months later, the news agency Reuters reported that Unicharm Corporation – Japan's market leader in adult incontinence products – was using a phrase in *its* advertising which translates as 'lil' dribble'. The Unicharm spokesman Hitoshi Watanabe said, 'What we are doing is trying to let people know that incontinence, even among young people, is normal.'[6]

If you've spent even a fraction of the time I have searching the internet for pelvic floor fixes, you'll no doubt already have heard that leaking is not, in fact, 'normal'. Common? Yes. Normal? No. It's an important distinction to make, because 'normal' implies that it's par for the course, and nothing to make a fuss about. It also implies that there's nothing to be done about it, even though, as we've heard, treatments are available – surgical and non-surgical –

which, for many, can help. There's every reason not to put up with it, yet so many people do. It will often take years to seek medical help – an average of seven, according to one poll.[7] And when asked by researchers in another study why they waited so long, women said they were worried about wasting the doctor's time, they were too embarrassed or too busy.[8]

Left untreated, these problems are unlikely to get better. If anything, they'll get worse. Take prolapse as an example. When researchers at the University of Stirling interviewed patients about their experiences of care, they made the point that when prolapse is detected early, conservative treatments like lifestyle changes and pelvic floor muscle training are more likely to be effective. But they found that women often delayed seeing a doctor because they were embarrassed or confused about their symptoms. When they did go, there was sometimes a lack of awareness among medical professionals, and women weren't always taken seriously until things got worse. 'By the time prolapse was suspected and a specialist referral made,' said Dr Purva Abhyankar, who led the study, 'the condition had progressed to the extent that surgery was the only viable option left.'[9]

We are great at putting ourselves last. And that's exactly where Rachel found herself. With three children and a busy career, she put on a pad and put up with incontinence, avoiding the things that made her leak. It was only when the marathon came up that she knew she had to try to do something about it. Rachel asked around surreptitiously. Had any of her friends had these kinds of issues? Did anybody know anybody who might be able to help? She was given a recommendation for a private physiotherapist, booked an appointment and suddenly found the space to unburden herself. I know this will resonate with many of you. When do we ever get a chance to really process our births? Or what comes after? It was as if a huge weight had been lifted:

> She just listened and then she said, "OK, we can fix this." And I burst into tears because I felt heard. And it's not that other people in my life weren't listening. I just wasn't talking because I didn't have the time or the space. I had so many other things and so many other people to look after before me.

Rachel had a lot of work to do. She embarked on an intensive training plan of squats, squeezes, lunges and weights, as well as using all the latest pelvic floor gadgets and gizmos (there is a whole world of delights which we'll get to later), all with the goal of getting the muscles of her entire core fighting fit. And she started to view her incontinence as an injury that needed to be fixed, not as an inevitable part of motherhood: 'If I had an Achilles injury, or if I had a shoulder injury which was stopping me from doing sport that I loved, I would do everything in my power to get that fixed, so why am I not fixing this injury?'

The first time it was suggested to me that pelvic floor dysfunction was an 'injury', it stopped me in my tracks. I hadn't thought about it in those terms before. To me, an injury was a cut or a broken bone, a burn or a strained muscle – serious wounds that happened suddenly and deserved proper treatment; things that could often be fixed. In my mind, that didn't include the likes of prolapse or incontinence or pelvic pain. I don't really know why. Maybe on some level I saw my own issues as insignificant or inevitable. As something I had brought on myself. I still struggle with it a bit. But I also see that if we can start to view these things as physical injuries, as wounds, then everything shifts. Because, as Rachel put it: 'It makes it seem less self-indulgent to try to fix it.'

Rachel spent eight years thinking incontinence was the price of having a family. Now she was realizing that it wasn't: 'There's a sense that wearing a pad or not being able to jump is almost a badge of honour – it's what we go through as women. And it's not. Having incontinence issues because you've had children, yes, it is part of the story, but you've got to get to the next chapter where you fix it. You don't just put up with it.'

All the hard work was paying off. Rachel was making progress. She no longer needed to wear pads every day and she could run three miles dry, for which she was incredibly grateful. Then, at the start of 2020, along came Covid, the world went into meltdown and the marathon was cancelled, but Rachel kept up the running. She had discovered a love for it. She had found freedom at a time when we were all locked down. She told me how liberating it was to be running through the woods near her home, sometimes while screaming out loud, much to the amusement of passers-by. I can absolutely relate as I jog around my local park with my headphones in. I haven't screamed yet, but when no one's looking I have been known to bust out a Phoebe Buffay-style run. I think it's fair to say that Rachel and I have found the mental health boost immeasurable.

The marathon was rescheduled for October 2021 and, in the months leading up to it, Rachel returned to training full pelt, but she was still leaking, especially on longer runs, ducking behind trees to change pads and feeling pretty miserable about it. So she went back to the GP and started using a bladder support or incontinence pessary, which you wear like a tampon to help stop urine escaping. Rachel calls it her 'sports bra' for her vagina and says it took a couple of weeks to pluck up the courage to use it, but, once she did, she noticed an improvement straight away.

Then, because nothing is ever straightforward, something unexpected happened. After months of working to strengthen her pelvic floor, Rachel was told the muscles were, in fact, too tight or 'hypertonic', sometimes described as 'overactive'. Wait, what? When I first came across this idea, it blew my mind. Surely that's the holy grail? Isn't this what we're all supposed to be working towards? But it isn't. The muscles have to be able to tighten *and* relax, because when they can't let go, when they're constantly on, they get too tired to work properly. And this can cause all kinds of symptoms, including constipation, pelvic pain, painful sex and, in Rachel's case, incontinence. She says working on that with a physiotherapist, using internal massage and a focus on relaxing the muscles, made an enormous difference.

Choosing to run a marathon is no small feat, not even for those in the best of health. Running puts a lot of pressure on the pelvic floor and is not something that should be taken lightly, especially if you already have pelvic floor problems. So, if you're thinking of doing it, please seek expert help. But it doesn't necessarily mean you can never run again. It doesn't have to be game over. Rachel understood that the marathon would take a huge toll on her body, and she knew she might not be able to run the whole thing dry. The real goal, though, was so much bigger than crossing the finish line. It was about recognizing that these injuries were not something to put up with or stay quiet about. It was about quality of life:

> I would love to do a five-mile run and, at the end of it, meet my husband and kids for coffee without having to firstly deal with a heavy wet pad, sodden leggings and, let's be honest, sometimes a bit of nappy rash. That's where I want to get to. If I can get to that I would be so proud of my body. To have recovered from going through the carrying and birth of three children, to run five miles dry, would be magical to me.

On the morning of 3 October 2021, Rachel lined up alongside 80,000 other runners in the autumn sunshine to take on the London Marathon. Four hours and fifty-four minutes later, she crossed the finish line, having run 26.2 miles *dry*.

Hypertonic Pelvic Floor

- The muscles of the pelvic floor must be able to contract *and* relax in order to properly function.
- A 'hypertonic' or 'overactive' pelvic floor is where the muscles of the pelvic floor become too tight and can't relax.
- Symptoms include pelvic pain, incontinence, constipation and painful sex.
- A pelvic health physiotherapist can assess you and help you learn to relax the muscles using pelvic floor exercise, deep breathing or internal massage.
- Don't just put up with it!

CHAPTER 8

EMMA

(MIND THE GAP)

I got an email once, describing the podcast as 'one of the best pieces of feminist broadcast on the internet'. I was pretty chuffed to read that, but also surprised. I wasn't really thinking big-picture when I started sharing stories about malfunctioning pelvic floors; I was just enraged that no one was talking about them, and I could see how damaging that was. The email went on to say (in capital letters) that 'PROLAPSE IS POLITICAL and the way that you're opening people's eyes to the insufficient care many women receive is so important.' I remember reading it on my phone in the kitchen and it stuck with me. It put into words something that I was feeling but had shied away from.

As I released more episodes and spoke to more women about their experiences, listeners were starting to join the dots, arguably faster than I was. Common themes were emerging around a lack of information and inadequate care and support, not just in the days and weeks around birth, but in the months and lifetimes that followed. There were more messages – people were telling me that 'the silence around these problems is a feminist issue' and that the podcast was 'exactly the sort of content the world needs more of if women's postpartum healthcare is ever going to be truly good enough'. At around the same time, I started hearing about the gender health gap – health inequalities that exist between male and female patients, deep-rooted inequalities that have been around for centuries. And it made me think that maybe I needed to get a bit more macro about this; that maybe you can't view pelvic floor dysfunction in isolation.

It's slowly being recognized that women's health has not been given the priority it deserves; that it's been underfunded and under-researched, and that it's led to many women receiving poorer healthcare than men. When the UK government announced plans for its first Women's Health Strategy for England in 2021, the then health secretary, Matt Hancock, put it in writing in the ministerial foreword: 'For generations, women have lived with a health and care system that is mostly designed by men, for men. This has meant that not enough is known about conditions that only affect women, or about how conditions that affect both men and women impact women in different ways. Pregnant women and women of childbearing age are also under-represented in clinical trials, which can create troubling gaps in data and understanding. This problem affects half of our population. It can lead to poorer advice and diagnosis and, as a result, worse outcomes.'[1]

The evidence is there, and it goes way beyond female-specific health needs like menopause or heavy periods. Research published by the House of Lords in 2021 pulls together studies and documents which show how women get a worse deal in all sorts of ways.[2] How they're more likely to experience common mental health conditions like anxiety or depression; how women with dementia are not as well monitored as men and take more potentially harmful medication; or how women who have heart attacks are more likely than men to *die*, because they're more likely to be misdiagnosed.[3,4,5]

Then there's the fact that women's pain is not always taken as seriously as men's. In 2008, researchers found that in US emergency departments, women in acute pain waited longer to be seen than men and were less likely to be given effective painkillers.[6] In another study, published in 2021 in the excellently named *Journal of Pain*, researchers at the University of Miami asked a group of observers to watch videos of people with shoulder injuries, and to judge how much pain they were in based on their facial expressions. When male and female patients expressed the same amount of pain, it was felt that females' pain was less intense. Not only that, but that they were more likely to benefit from psychotherapy than from medication; essentially, that it was all in their head.[7] The research was co-authored by Elizabeth Losin, assistant professor of psychology and director of the Social and Cultural Neuroscience lab at the University of Miami, who said: 'If the stereotype is to think women are more expressive than men, perhaps "overly" expressive, then the tendency will be to discount women's pain behaviours. The flip side of this stereotype is that men are perceived to be stoic, so when a man makes an intense pain facial expression, you think, "Oh my, he must be dying!"'[8]

Women are not being heard when it comes to health, and sometimes with devastating consequences. In 2020, an independent inquiry looked at how the healthcare system in England responds when patients report harmful side effects from medicines and medical devices. The Cumberlege Review found that women had suffered 'avoidable harm' because they weren't listened to, sometimes for decades. The review focused on three interventions: two medicines which, when taken during pregnancy, are thought to be linked to birth defects (hormonal pregnancy tests and the epilepsy drug, sodium valproate), and pelvic (or vaginal) mesh, an implant used to treat incontinence and prolapse, which can have serious complications, with thousands of women reporting life-changing injuries. The stories are heartbreaking: women in chronic pain who have lost their mobility, independence, careers and sex lives; women who weren't warned of the risks and weren't listened to when things went wrong. The report criticized the healthcare system for 'a culture of dismissive and arrogant attitudes', where symptoms were labelled as 'normal' or put down to 'women's problems'.

I sometimes hear from women who have come up against outrageous attitudes in healthcare – not just dismissive or arrogant, but sexist, misogynist even. Like the woman who was told by a doctor that wearing a pessary would be like putting a mousetrap in her husband's 'play pen'. She was dumbstruck. And too embarrassed to complain. Of course, not every medical professional is like that. Let's hope they are few and far between. But it's not the first time I've come across this sort of exchange.

Conscious or unconscious, the gender bias in health is real, and sometimes it's compounded by other inequalities. Let's not forget that black women in the UK are still more than four times as likely as white women to die in pregnancy or childbirth; or that women in the most deprived parts of England are dying eight years sooner than those in the wealthiest areas; or that LGBT+ people report poorer health than the general population and worse experiences of healthcare.[10,11,12] Thankfully, there are brilliant researchers, journalists and campaigners who are shining a light on all of this. One of them is Sarah Graham, a health journalist and founder of the *Hysterical Women* blog, which explores women's experiences of sexism and dismissal in healthcare. When we sat down to record in 2022, she was writing her book *Rebel Bodies: A guide to the gender health gap revolution*, and she told me how that gap manifests in lots of different ways, some more obvious than others:

> Sometimes it's just the really insidious things you think nothing of at the time – like a GP that's a little bit dismissive when you go to them with something that actually is having quite a big impact on your life, all the way through to the much, much bigger things, like women not getting the care they need for the really serious, potentially life-

threatening issues. It's massive. And once you're aware of it . . . you see it everywhere.

It's true. Once you get your head around how wild it is, you can't stop seeing it. And one of the big factors in all of it is a lack of research or, more specifically, a lack of research involving women; we simply don't know enough about female bodies, so we don't know how to treat them. My mind was blown when I read Caroline Criado Perez's book, *Invisible Women: Exposing data bias in a world designed for men*. The writer and campaigner argues that, for thousands of years, men have been seen as the default in pretty much every aspect of life, and she points to study after jaw-dropping study that demonstrate how the world has been designed around that. She explains how the male body is seen as the 'norm', including when it comes to medicine, leaving women more or less absent from the medical textbooks and routinely under-represented in clinical trials, and not just women, but female animals and even cells too. All of it contributing to a medical system which, she says, 'from root to tip, is systemically discriminating against women, leaving them chronically misunderstood, mistreated and misdiagnosed'.[13]

And it's not just that women are missing from the data. When it comes to conditions that mostly affect women, the data is often missing altogether. Endometriosis is held up as a common example. It's a disease where tissue similar to the lining of the womb grows elsewhere in the body.

It can be very painful, it can cause infertility and, according to the World Health Organization, it affects one in ten women of reproductive age.[14] Yet, in 2020, a report by MPs found that there's been so little investment in research that we don't know what causes it, let alone have a cure, and that, on average, it takes eight years to even get a diagnosis.[15]

I see it now. All of this is going on in the background when you try to navigate pelvic floor problems after babies – when you are fobbed off or told it's 'normal'; when you struggle to be taken seriously; or when you can't find information or access the treatment you deserve. Maybe it goes some way towards explaining why there aren't better treatments in the first place. It's a subject that the broadcaster and journalist Emma Barnett is no stranger to.

It took twenty-one years for Emma to get a diagnosis for endometriosis – two decades of what she describes as 'bone-grinding pain' and then fertility issues. She'd been to the GP, repeatedly, but it took a friend who was an obstetrician to finally piece it all together. Emma shared her story in her book *It's About Bloody Time. Period*, smashing all the stigmas about menstruation and exploding all the myths (and somehow managing to be funny at the same time). She eventually had a child through IVF, but says she still 'survives' the disease, and she's vocal about it. She writes articles, she campaigns and she does it all with zero embarrassment. She had no qualms whatsoever about unwittingly becoming the first person to announce on live TV that she was menstruating, or that it was really hurting. For Emma, talking about gynae issues has never been a problem.

But here's the thing: despite being more clued up than most of us about gynaecological health, and despite being fearless when it comes to discussing it, Emma was completely in the dark when she, like Rachel, went on to develop a tight pelvic floor – where the muscles are too tense, just constantly contracting. She told me it was one of the 'most upsetting' things she's ever been through. And it's why I wanted to speak to her on the podcast. Because if an award-winning journalist with this kind of insight struggles to access the information or help she needs, what hope is there for the rest of us?

Emma and I used to work for the same radio network and she once presented a discussion about pelvic floor dysfunction, which I produced. Somewhere in the middle of that she very briefly mentioned that she had this 'hypertonic' pelvic floor, and I couldn't let that slide. Emma is another one who seemingly never stops – if she's not broadcasting or writing or parenting, then she's public-speaking or hosting – but I finally managed to catch up with her, not long after she started a new job presenting the institution that is *Woman's Hour* on BBC Radio 4. Emma lives in London but is a proud Mancunian and, when we spoke, she had just got home from work and changed into a T-shirt with 'Buzzin' R Kid' plastered across the front. As a fellow northerner, I very much approved.

This was the first time Emma had spoken in detail about

what happened and she told me she was doing it because she didn't want other people to go through what she had. She said that things began to unravel around three months after her son was born by caesarean. She didn't know the first thing about pelvic floors, but she had a horrible tense feeling that she just couldn't shake and she found herself scrabbling around on the internet late at night, wondering if she was losing her mind: 'It felt like I was holding my breath, in my body. And I don't know if I'm explaining that well, but I just couldn't relax my pelvic floor. I couldn't bring it down. I mean obviously you're stressed when you're a new mum and you're trying to figure stuff out, but even when I was relaxed and it was all quite chilled, I couldn't get this thing to go down.'

It was painful too, really painful, and it all came to a head a few weeks later, just hours before a big political interview. Emma told me she was getting ready to guest-present what was *The Andrew Marr Show* – a Sunday morning politics programme on BBC One. It was her first shift back at work and she was due to interview the UK Culture Secretary, so she was going through it all with her producers – Brexit policy and Labour's position on it, how the government was going to launch a paper on online safety – but she was struggling: 'I was trying to get my head around some quite complicated things, and all I could think about was my bloody pelvic floor. And I said to myself, if I get through the next twenty-four hours workwise, I'm going to make myself a promise that I will see somebody about this.'

Emma got through the day, but finding somebody to see about it was a challenge in itself. She didn't know who to talk to, and the whole thing seemed so shrouded in secrecy that even looking it up felt weird, 'clandestine' almost. She was desperate for a diagnosis, but NHS waiting lists were endless and the health insurer she spoke to didn't even know how to categorize it. It wasn't until she finally managed to find her way to a private pelvic health physiotherapist that she began to understand what was happening – that she had this hypertonic pelvic floor:

> She said, "It's really bad but not as bad as I've seen, so you're lucky." And I thought, "Oh my gosh, it could be worse?" And I'm getting quite emotional even thinking back to this, because I was lying on the table and it was the first time I'd been apart from my son for a long period of time, and I don't know if it was because it was to do with him and his birth, but I thought, "Am I ever going to be normal again?"

Emma told me that physiotherapy 'saved' her. She was shown techniques to help relax her pelvic floor – exercises and breath work which helped to calm everything down. She had to work at it, she still does. Sometimes it's better and sometimes it's all-consuming; at least now she knows what it is, how to manage it and where to go when she needs help. But she said she's scared for women who don't have that help, and that it's 'not acceptable' that, in Britain, postpartum care barely exists. Emma's sister-in-law had one of her children in France where, as we've heard, women's physio is a standard part of recovery. 'Well, why don't we have that? Can we please just agree that we need a bit of aftercare when we've done the equivalent of a marathon in our body once a day for nine months?'

You'd be hard-pushed to find a mum who would disagree. In England, at around six weeks after giving birth, you're supposed to have a physical and mental check with a doctor, separate to the baby's six-week check. Since April 2020, and the Covid pandemic aside, GPs have been *required* to offer this, which is a good thing, but it's a ten-minute appointment at best, and it's meant to put you back together after one of the most physical and emotional events of your life, so, with the best will in the world, with the best GP in the world, it's never going to be sufficient. They'll inquire about your mental health, which, of course, is hugely important, but a thorough check of your pelvic floor is not on the agenda – if you're lucky you might be asked about it or advised to do your Kegels.

When I asked on Instagram for recent experiences of the 'six-week check', one woman told me she steeled herself to *request* a physical exam, only to be told by her GP that he 'wouldn't know what he was looking at'. Another summed it up as, 'contraception and crack on' because, for reasons that are far from obvious to me, there's often this relentless focus on birth control, as if a shredded perineum or major surgery isn't contraception enough. I'm yet to meet a mum who doesn't roll her eyes at this, not least because, the last time I checked, family planning was not solely a female responsibility. Some women told me they hadn't been offered an appointment at all, others that it was on the phone but they were at least asked about their pelvic floor, which is all to say that what we have is a start, but it's nowhere near enough.

None of this is about knocking overworked or under-resourced health professionals. The NHS is filled with hard-working, passionate and dedicated staff who are often doing an impossible job under enormous pressure. I'm hugely grateful to live in a country with a publicly funded healthcare system that is universal, and free at the point of need. But it doesn't always work. Services don't always meet the need. Patients don't always get the care they deserve. And what this is about is the bigger picture – long-term change, from the top. What gets prioritized and what doesn't, *who* gets prioritized and who doesn't.

Conversations are happening. When the UK government asked for experiences to inform its Women's Health Strategy, it was inundated with more than 100,000 replies. Women said that they didn't feel listened to by some health professionals, that they didn't feel supported. You can hear it loud and clear in a short film on the BBC News website. Three women are chatting about their health conditions at a hairdresser's: they talk about delays in diagnosis and treatment and how they were told that heavy and painful periods were 'just bad luck'. One woman says she wasn't offered enough support when she discovered that she had a prolapse. 'Let's face it,' says another, 'you've either got a vagina or a voice. You don't seem to have both, do you?'[16]

In response to the public consultation, the government appointed a dedicated women's health ambassador for England and, in July 2022, published its long-awaited plan for change, a 127-page document promising to 'improve the way in which the health and care system listens to women's voices, and boost health outcomes for women and girls'.[17]

The way I see it, any acknowledgement that women are getting a worse deal on health, simply because of who they are, is welcome. That alone, I hope, will drive change. In terms of the ten-year plan, a few things stood out to me, like the fact that, from 2024, all *new* doctors will have mandatory training and assessment on women's health (I know, it's hard to believe it wasn't happening already); that women's health hubs are going to be 'encouraged' (where existing services are brought together under one roof); that the NHS website will have its content on women's health updated; and that there'll be investment in research into women's health, as well as better representation of women in research more generally. There are questions about how this long list of ambitions will be funded, but the consensus seems to be that it's a start.

There are similar plans being put in place to improve women's health across the rest of the UK, so the acknowledgement is there, and some action is being taken. Whether we'll notice a significant change remains to be seen. 'It's really tricky,' said Sarah Graham when I asked her about it, 'because it is so deeply ingrained. There's no one thing that would fix the whole problem – no amount of money and research and training, as brilliant as all that stuff is. It all has to come together and it's going to take a really long time to shift the culture and change attitudes, but I'm fairly hopeful that things are going in the right direction.'

I don't know if it's helpful or not to have all of this in the back of your mind as you try to manage your pelvic floor problems, but it's fascinating to me, and I think important if we want things to change. Maybe it's given you some rage and maybe that's no bad thing, because sometimes anger can help you stand your ground, to make some noise and demand better treatment. It can help you advocate for yourself or even just tell someone how you feel. Emma's advice is to 'tool yourself up' with as much information as you can, and then to write it all down or share it with someone you trust, so that you know you can articulate it. 'And then,' she told me, 'the real work begins, of trying to see somebody and actually get some treatment. Treat it like a full project, like a full-time thing, even if you can't do it full-time, because there's nothing more important than your health.'

The Gender Health Gap

- The gender health gap describes health inequalities that exist between male and female patients.
- The UK government has acknowledged that, historically, the health and care system has been 'designed by men, for men'.[18]
- England's first ever Women's Health Strategy was launched in July 2022, promising to 'reset the dial' on women's health, with similar plans announced in Scotland and Wales.
- Do your research, and don't be afraid to advocate for yourself. As Emma said, 'There's nothing more important than your health.'

CHAPTER 9

GAYNOR

(PESSARIES AND 'VADGETS')

The first time I tried a vaginal pessary it fell out in the hospital car park. I'd been fitted with a ring to help support my pelvic organs, but the journey out of the building was enough to dislodge it; I don't mean it was rolling around on the road, nothing as dramatic or entertaining as that, but it wasn't staying in. Pessaries are medical devices that are meant to sit inside the vagina and hold everything in place, but it turns out they don't come in a one-size-fits-all and there's often a bit (or sometimes a lot) of trial and error involved. They don't work for everybody either, but when they do, they can make all the difference. One listener told me how wearing one has meant she's been able to run for the first time in six years; another, that it's working so well she's postponed surgery, 'indefinitely'.

This is not revolutionary technology. If you had a prolapse in Greece a couple of thousand years ago, you might have been prescribed a pomegranate as a pessary – chopped in half and soaked in vinegar.[1] Or you might have been tied to a wooden frame by your feet, shaken violently up and down, and left in bed for three days with your legs bound together (don't try this at home), so, on balance, maybe fruit was not such a bad option. Over the years, pessaries have become more durable, with pomegranates replaced by cork, wood or brass, then later glass and porcelain. Thankfully, these days they're usually made of plastic or silicone, and they come in a mind-boggling range of shapes and sizes, not just the standard-issue NHS ring. There are cubes, ovals, doughnuts, dishes, shelves and many more. Some you can wear during intercourse, others you can't; some you take in and out every day, others you can leave in for months at a time. You can also get bladder support pessaries, which are specifically for incontinence. You get the idea.

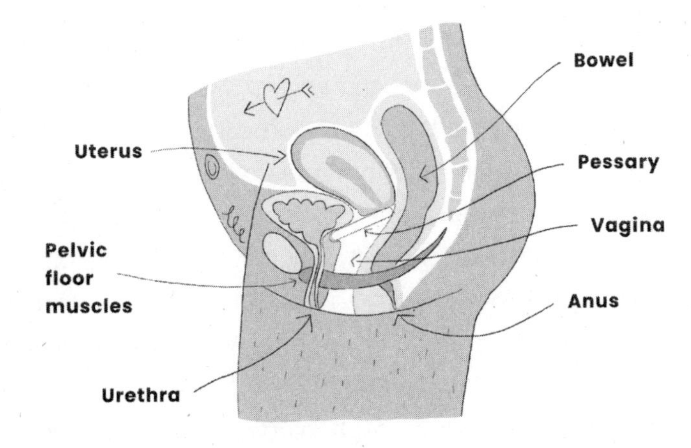

Despite being around for millennia, it won't surprise you that I had never heard of a pessary before I was a candidate for one, and that even afterwards I struggled to understand what was available or what might work. I don't know why the information isn't easier to find, but whenever pessaries are mentioned on the podcast, I get a ton of questions. How do you get one in and out? Can you wear one in pregnancy? How long does it last? Can you wear one with a coil? There's confusion about what's available, and how to manage it, and where to go in the first place. You're back to playing the old postcode lottery of finding someone to prescribe one. Some GPs do it, some nurse practitioners, some consultants and some physios. Some will have different styles and brands available, others will have a drawer full of rings and nothing more. Some will fit them, others won't. You might wait a few weeks, or you might wait a year. It's a very mixed picture and expertise seems scarce. If I had a pound for every woman who's been wrongly told by a doctor that they're 'too young' for a pessary, I'd be rich; even though it's there in black and white in the NICE guidelines as a first-line treatment for prolapse, and something to consider for incontinence too, after lifestyle changes and pelvic floor muscle training.[2] It makes no sense to me. Not least because what happens then is that some women go online and buy their own, without any advice or guidance, which, for obvious reasons, is far from ideal.

Pessaries aside, there's an ever-growing arsenal of pelvic floor gadgets available which, collectively, I like to call 'vadgets' in the vague hope it will catch on. It's another wildly confusing landscape to navigate, and includes weights, electrical stimulators, biofeedback machines, apps and even video games (because, why not?), all designed to help train your pelvic floor. It's a bit overwhelming, to say the least. Who are they for? How do they work? Do they work? It's why I wanted to speak to the pelvic health physiotherapist and self-described gadget nerd, Amanda Savage, who carried out a review of a huge range of devices. When I recorded with her (and her dog, Tilly), she told me that, for some people, with the right guidance, they can be really effective: 'I think one of the reasons that gadgets can work is because they make you stop still and actually do it properly. If you've gone to all the effort to take your kit off and put something inside and plug into a machine, you're not going to just drift off and put a wash on, are you?'

I think you can see why I like Amanda. And she knows her stuff. She helpfully broke everything down into categories, starting with **electrical stimulators**, which your physio might recommend if your pelvic floor muscles are so weak you can barely feel them. They usually consist of an internal probe, which is hooked up to a machine and passes a small electrical current through the muscles to make them contract and relax. They basically do the work for you, until you get to a point where you can do it yourself. I suggested to Amanda that the idea of putting an electrical probe in your vagina sounded slightly terrifying, but she told me it shouldn't be: 'I think if you can remember that that's what your brain does – that's what nature does. Nature sends an electrical pulse from your brain to your pelvic floor, and what we're doing with these devices is to kind of skip the brain out and to take a more direct route.'

Biofeedback is the term for another group of gadgets

which tell you if you're doing your pelvic floor exercises correctly; a bit of visual motivation, if you like. I was once given a biofeedback device called 'The Educator', which made me smile because I thought it sounded more like a wrestler than a piece of medical kit. It's a little white plastic probe with a stick on a hinge, which rises and falls as you squeeze and relax your pelvic floor muscles. It sounds bizarre and it is, but it gets way more bizarre than that. And way more high-tech. You can get biofeedback devices which, instead of a stick, give you a reading on a screen. When you squeeze, they send the information to a machine, or wirelessly, to an app on your phone. And yes, this is where you can use your pelvic floor muscles to play actual video games – shooting virtual basketball hoops, controlling bubbles or flying around collecting things as a butterfly or an octopus. I've yet to try this, but it's definitely on my bucket list, out of curiosity if nothing else.

You can get other **apps** too, which remind you to do your pelvic floor exercises and help you to stay on track. They tend to have a visual timer you can follow as you squeeze, which stops you from rushing, and these don't come with an internal probe, so there's no need to get half-naked – you can Kegel anytime, anywhere. Then, as a low-tech option, there are **vagina weights or cones**; just another thing that made me double-take when I first heard about them, and which might be recommended if you need the extra challenge. You're supposed to use your pelvic floor muscles to hold them inside, but maybe stay close to home when you do it: 'They do infer that you could wear your weights to Sainsbury's or the gym,' Amanda explained, 'but I've never really thought that was a terribly good idea – I'm not really for ultimate risk. Personally, I've always advised that you make it a focused task, in your own home, and I usually suggest something like when you wash your hair in the shower.'

The list of devices available to help train your pelvic floor is seemingly endless. Google it and you'll see what I mean. As for how effective they are, the committee behind the new NICE guidelines says that some studies do show benefits, but that, once again, more evidence is needed.[3] Amanda told me that, for some people, they can work, but they should be used under the guidance of a medical professional, and they need to be part of what you're doing, not the only thing you're doing:

> Just sitting at home, stimulating your pelvic floor with a device will not be enough. You've also got to get your core working, you've got to look at your bladder habits, you've got to think about your lifting and carrying and you've got to teach your brain to do that job when you're not plugged into a machine.

Demand is certainly there. Sales of 'vadgets' are rising globally. The market for pelvic floor stimulators alone was valued at US$180 million in 2020 and is forecast to more than double by 2028 – driven in part by a growing awareness of

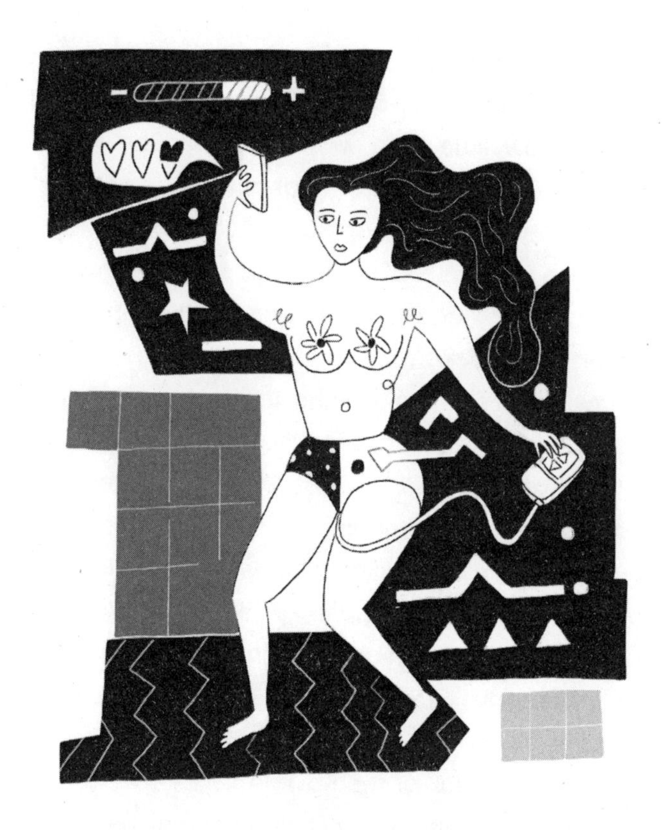

women's health, an ageing population and the development of new technology.[4] And it's not just pelvic floor devices that are seeing a boost, there are a growing number of apps, products and services addressing *other* female-specific health needs, including menstruation, fertility and menopause. 'Femtech' is booming, a sector that didn't even exist in 2013, when Dr Tania Boler co-founded the technology brand, Elvie, to address neglected issues in women's health.

Tania became passionate about pelvic health when she

was pregnant. She was shocked to discover just how common it was to experience conditions like incontinence and prolapse, and how little help was available. She went on to develop the Elvie Trainer, a biofeedback device that connects to an app on your phone. I'm sure you've seen it – a sort of pastel-green egg with a curved tail, but way more stylish than I've made it sound. It was a hard sell though. She's since spoken about how the taboo made it difficult to find investment, how it was seen as a 'niche' topic and how, in the early days, people didn't take it seriously. She got there in the end, and Elvie has become one of Europe's fastest growing companies. Its latest product is a wearable breast pump, which made headlines when it launched in 2018, worn by a model on the catwalk at London Fashion Week. But in spite of the buzz around it, Tania says this kind of technology is *still* a hard sell. She spoke to the *Financial Times* in September 2021: 'I think we're still having to justify and explain the size of the problem with the lack of tech available for women's health. And we have to continually say this is not a niche market and these are real issues, even if they're hidden.'[5]

The way I see it, the more we talk about it, the more the world will see that these are not 'niche' issues, and the more investors and decision makers will sit up and take notice. Maybe that will lead to better treatments or better care. And the innovators are out there – they always have been. Gaynor Morgan is a pelvic health advocate and educator, known as Pelvic Angel. I invited her on the podcast as a pessary expert – it was going to be a how-to guide, an entire episode dedicated to what's what and debunking some myths. But then I heard the most incredible story about how she came to invent her own pessary after seeing her mum suffer with incontinence, and I had to ask her about it. It begins in the eighties, on the south coast of Wales where Gaynor grew up. She and her mum, Carole, were really close, more like best friends than mother and daughter. There were only seventeen years between them, and they would hit the discos of Swansea together, dancing to Soft Cell and loving life.

Gaynor told me that her mum was cheerful and outgoing, but she had stress incontinence, where you leak when you cough, sneeze or exercise. Surgery helped for a while, but it got worse again as time went on, and by her mid-forties it was affecting her confidence as well as intimacy with her partner. She stopped going out, ended the relationship and became depressed and withdrawn. She was so embarrassed that it got to the point where she rarely left the house. At one stage, she wanted to take her own life because of it; and when she went to see her GP, she was told she was too heavy for more surgery, given some antidepressants and sent on her way.

Gaynor was working overseas by then, so it was only when she came home on leave that she saw how bad things were. She started searching around for something, anything, that might help her mum. She remembers sitting on the sofa one day when Carole mentioned that the leaking stopped during her period, when she was wearing a tampon. They were both trained nurses and it didn't take long for them to work out what was happening. 'We looked at the anatomy side of it and thought, "Gosh, it's that simple. This tampon is compressing against the urethra and that's what's stopping the involuntary loss of urine."' Carole started wearing a tampon when she wasn't menstruating, with a condom over the top to prevent infection, and it stopped the leaks. They wanted to tell the world. They wrote to the tampon manufacturer saying, '"Do you know what? If you dip this in latex, you are going to have an amazing product to stop women leaking." You can imagine, they must have thought we were a couple of fruitcakes.' Ignored but unperturbed, they decided to invent their own.

They made a mould using odds and ends they found around the house – air-dry clay from a child's craft project, a candle, a McDonald's straw and a key ring . . . I'm not kidding. Then they filled it with liquid latex and, when it dried, they had something that looked like a tampon with a stem on it. Carole started using that, again with a condom over it, and again it worked. Gaynor laughed when she told me that the news spread like wildfire around the little Welsh village where they lived, and where she said everybody knew everything: 'If you farted in the wrong direction, Mrs Jones down the road would soon complain. So we had women knocking on the door going, "Can we have one of these products?" and we were quite happily making them in the kitchen, not realizing that there could have been a lawsuit around the corner because they could have caused some kind of damage to somebody.'

It was a chance conversation with Carole's gynaecologist that led to a more serious proposition. One meeting led to another; and mother and daughter started developing, researching and tackling the red tape, trailing around medical fairs to find the best materials, getting the right permissions and preparing for clinical trials. It took more than ten years, but eventually their home-made prototype became 'Inco-Stress' – an incontinence pessary that sits in the vagina and supports the bladder and urethra. Tragically, Carole died suddenly in 2004, before the trials were published, and when she was just fifty-nine years old. Gaynor was devastated, but she knew she had to push through and bring the device to market: 'I thought, "I can either spiral into the wine bottle or I can pull my finger out of my backside, move forward and help as many people as I can."' So she moved forward.

The trials took place at Gaynor's local hospital and were a success: 30 per cent of those who took part came off the waiting list for surgery, preferring to use the pessary instead. Gaynor opened the business in her mum's memory, and it went from strength to strength, winning awards and gaining momentum globally. She still gets letters from women around the world, thanking her for helping them to live a more normal life, to exercise, to run around with their kids and regain their self-confidence. It's not a silver bullet, but it's another tool in the armoury.

After the car park incident, I tried a couple of other ring pessaries and found one that stayed in. I wore it for several months, but it didn't seem to make any difference to my symptoms, and I wanted to see how I would be without it, so I had it removed. It was only when I started making the podcast and having more conversations about what was available that I considered trying again. I was hearing success stories and I started to wonder if a different style would work. What if I could learn to manage it myself? Maybe it could give me some control over my symptoms, some protection from things getting worse.

It took me ages to get around to making an appointment. I kept saying I would and then I didn't. It occurred to me afterwards that I was putting it off in case it didn't work. That I'd been 'saving it' for if or when my symptoms got worse. I wanted to know that I had something in reserve, that there was something else I could try if I really needed it. I'm sure there's some logic in there somewhere. I did call the GP eventually, got a referral, and waited. And waited. I was still waiting almost a year later, when I received an offer that I couldn't refuse. A women's health physiotherapist, Tracey Matthews, had been following my story on Instagram and offered me a pessary fitting at a private clinic in London. I was there over Easter visiting family, so it made sense to go for it.

Tracey offered to let me record the fitting for the podcast, to give some insight into how it works, and I filmed a bit too, for social media. I know how strange that sounds and, trust me, no one is more surprised than I am, but lots of unusual things have happened since I started all of this and now I'm just rolling with it.

Tracey also has first-hand experience of prolapse, which she developed after her son was born. She went through *all* the emotions, but as a former GB rower and a weightlifter, she knew she had to find a way back to fitness, so pessaries became her thing. She trained to fit them, and she wears one too – for lifting and for running. She told me it's not an easy road, and her rehab involves a lot of pelvic floor training as well as whole-body strengthening, but that it's doable. And it's worth it: 'Prolapse doesn't have to be this devastating thing that you see on the internet. We can manage it. We don't have to accept it, we don't have to put up with it, and if pessaries help to take away that nagging symptom of just feeling it day to day, then why wouldn't we use them?'

Tracey cleared her diary to help me and I was there for a good couple of hours. She talked through my medical history, about where I wanted to get to, and she examined me and fitted me with a cube pessary, which looks like a large dice (some are larger than others) with rounded corners. It sits in the vagina to hold everything up and stays in place using suction, a bit like a menstrual cup. Then she sent me off for a brisk walk to make sure it didn't fall out and talked me through the pelvic floor training I should be doing to make sure I have the muscle bulk to support it. That part of the conversation can be summed up as 'must do better', but I left feeling really happy, hopeful that this little cube could be the support I needed to just get on with life.

I wish I could tell you that it was a miracle cure, but, in truth, I'm still experimenting. You think it fits and then you sit, stand, walk, visit the loo, and it shifts out of place. It could be the size. It could be that I need to bulk up the muscles. It could just not be for me. Tracey recommended that I keep my NHS appointment, which finally came through a few weeks later, and the specialist nurse there was wonderful too. Not only did she give me a couple of other sizes to try, but at one point she and the healthcare assistant joined me in bobbing up and down, jiggling and dancing around a tiny consultation room to check that the pessary that I was wearing didn't dislodge. Obviously, I was the only person in the room that needed to take part in that strange ritual, but I appreciated the support.

I don't know how it's all going to pan out, but I understand that, if I want it to work, I need to keep up with my pelvic floor training as well as strength training more generally. And, as I have already confessed, lately, for lots of reasons, I just haven't. Self-care has fallen down my personal list of priorities, but I'll get back to it. I haven't given up. As Gaynor pointed out, it was never going to be a quick fix: 'You know our vaginas are as unique as our thumbprints. There isn't going to be one pessary that's going to fix everybody. I can't see it happening in my lifetime. But there are companies out there that are continuously working on different methods, shapes and everything. Innovation doesn't stop.'

As I write, a company in Canada, Cosm Medical, is working on a way to make *customized* pessaries for prolapse. It involves using an ultrasound scan, artificial intelligence and 3D printing techniques to make a bespoke mould. I don't pretend to understand the technology behind it, but I wanted to find out a bit more, so I got on a video call with the founder and CEO, Derek Sham. He told me he started the company after his grandmother was diagnosed with late-stage prolapse. Her symptoms were debilitating, and conservative treatments didn't work. She ended up with an infection and, after several rounds of failed surgeries, was admitted to a care home because of it. It was heartbreaking for Derek, an engineer whose background is in urodynamics – tests for incontinence that assess how the bladder and urethra are performing. 'I knew some of the best doctors in the world,' he said, 'but I really couldn't get her the care that I thought she deserved.' It's what drove him to launch Cosm, in the hope that other women could be diagnosed and treated much sooner. He said he wants to change the standard of care for pelvic floor disorders, to get to a place where doctors don't have to rely on finger measurements as a diagnostic tool, which makes a lot of sense when you think about it. And if there's a chance that couture pessaries are going to become the next big thing, then I'm here for it.

Pessaries and 'Vadgets'

- A vaginal pessary is a removable medical device made of plastic or silicone.
- It sits in the vagina and can help you to manage prolapse by supporting the pelvic organs and holding them in place.
- There's a range of shapes, makes and sizes and they can be worn at any age.
- You can also get bladder support pessaries, for urinary incontinence.
- There's a growing number of pelvic floor gadgets (vadgets) designed to help train your pelvic floor (for example, electrical stimulators, biofeedback, weights or apps).
- Consult your GP or pelvic health physio if you're thinking of trying any of the above!

CHAPTER 10

JAN

(THE M WORD)

Pelvic floor problems don't always reveal themselves in the weeks and months after childbirth, sometimes they turn up years later, when your hormones change around (shhhh) menopause. Actually, we don't have to whisper it anymore – not since the menopause revolution began in all its noisy and unapologetic glory. Now it seems you can't move for books, campaigns or Davina McCall's giant billboard, and it's wonderful – this realization that, when half the planet goes through an inevitable and transformational physical change, we should probably talk about it. This is yet another thing that leaves you scratching your head and wondering how it hasn't happened before now.

The 'M' word has gone mainstream and it gives me hope, considering that just a few years ago it was so taboo that it was barely on our collective radar; it certainly wasn't on mine. I remember walking home after the school run one day and chatting to a friend who told me she thought she might be perimenopausal. Peri-what? We were still recovering from having babies and now we could be transitioning towards menopause? Cut us some slack.

Before then, what I thought I knew about menopause

amounted to this: it happened in your fifties, you got hot flushes, you cried a lot and your periods stopped; which I suppose is true for some, but it can be so much more than that. I went to a talk about menopause-in-the-workplace, where a senior police officer described how perimenopause had turned her life upside down at the age of forty-six. I sat there, wide-eyed, as she spoke about how she was completely unprepared when a combination of anxiety, brain fog and disturbed sleep made every day a struggle, affected her relationship and nearly drove her out of her dream job. Then she gave a long list of other potential symptoms to look out for, and it made my head swim. It included joint aches, irregular periods, weight gain, palpitations, reduced sex drive, mood changes, sweats, irritability, vaginal dryness and, of course, pelvic floor problems. I learned that fifty-one is the *average* age for actual menopause – a single day in your life that marks twelve months since your last period – but that all of this other stuff can be going on for months or for years before that.

It took a while, but I realized that I should probably take my head out of the sand, not least because I have a vested interest. I'm forty-three now and I already have a prolapse, so am I just doomed? Will it automatically get worse? It's a question I put to Michelle Lyons when I spoke to her for the podcast in January 2022. She's a women's health physiotherapist of nearly thirty years who educates other healthcare providers about menopause and has qualifications in yoga, Pilates, mindfulness and nutrition. And the good news is, she told me we're not doomed: 'Not at all, because knowledge is power.'

Michelle described perimenopause as a 'hormonal rollercoaster ride', which is different for everyone. It can last for ten years (or more) in the run-up to menopause and can lead to any number of physical and mental symptoms. In simple terms, she said a lot of those issues can be explained by a drop in oestrogen, a hormone which does hundreds of things in the female body including helping to regulate your menstrual cycle and maintain brain, bone and heart health. It's also important for your pelvic health because it helps to keep your muscles and ligaments strong and elastic, as well as plumping up the tissues around the openings in the pelvic floor (the urethra, anus and vagina), so when levels fall, it can contribute to incontinence, painful sex, prolapse, and so on, and sometimes expose problems that have been lying dormant for years.

> What can happen is maybe some of the issues that we developed after we had our babies come back, and say, "Hello, remember me? I haven't quite gone away and now that there's no oestrogen, let's talk about leaky bladders, bowel leakage and pelvic organ prolapse."

I have to be honest, it's not the most attractive prospect, but Michelle reassured me that we shouldn't despair – that it's all 'figureoutable'. For pelvic floors specifically, she said pelvic floor muscle training can sometimes be enough to manage milder issues, and that a lot of the more general symptoms can be helped with diet and lifestyle changes – all of the things we already know we should be doing, like eating well, sleeping well, managing stress and exercising. She said constipation is one of her 'topics of obsession', and is important for lots of reasons, like the fact that it can make incontinence worse, and because straining isn't great for your pelvic floor, but also because a happy gut is good for your hormone balance. And she knows it can sometimes be a 'hard pill to swallow', but for some, scaling back on alcohol might help too, because it can trigger symptoms and disrupt sleep.

There's something else you hear a lot about when it comes to managing menopause and perimenopause, and that's the importance of strength training – exercise that involves body weight or equipment to build muscle mass and strength – like yoga, or using free weights or resistance bands. That's because there's evidence that it helps not just with muscle health, but also bone and heart health, which is useful when falling oestrogen levels are having the opposite effect, but confusing if you have pelvic floor problems and have been advised, as we've heard, to avoid lifting.[1,2] We're back to The Fear around exercise and movement, but arguably at an even more important time in your life. Michelle's view, though, is that strength training is possible for everybody, and not just possible but 'vital' around menopause:

> Strength training means that if you're going to lift something heavy, you've got strong arms and legs to do

> the power of the move, and you're not holding your breath and bearing down on your poor old pelvic floor, and maybe putting your bladder or your prolapse under a little bit of pressure. It's suitable for everybody, it's just having this graded approach that you start where you are and then you find somebody to work with who can progress you through.

Michelle explained that, armed with the right knowledge and guidance, there's a lot you can do by yourself, but sometimes you'll need more help. You might see a pelvic health physio or ask a GP for specialist treatment. You might also decide to try hormone replacement therapy (HRT), which she said 'can be the boat that gets you to the other side'. HRT works by topping up hormone levels that have dipped as you approach menopause, and it's not the medical pariah it was twenty years ago. Prescription rates fell around the world in 2002 when the results of a major study linking it to breast cancer and heart disease were misreported. For years afterwards, women (and doctors) were understandably wary, but there's been a lot more research since then, and the current advice is that, for most women, the benefits of HRT outweigh the risks.[3] It won't be right for everyone; it's a discussion to have with your GP, but Michelle told me that it *can* help: 'We've really seen an explosion in the discussion around hormone therapy, and for women it can be an absolute game changer. It's not a magic bullet that you can use by yourself, but it can be a really good adjunct to helping women feel better.'

Of course, not everyone will need help. Some people get through it all pretty much unscathed. But for those who do struggle, the impact of perimenopause and menopause can't be overstated. Three-quarters of those who responded to a survey for the British Menopause Society said it had 'caused them to change their lives'. More than half said it had a 'negative' effect – on work, relationships and socializing.[4] And for years, women have been reporting that when they do go to the doctor, their symptoms are not recognized as menopause or that they're not taken seriously.[5] (Sound familiar?) In 2022 a report by MPs highlighted another 'postcode lottery' of specialist healthcare, where access to services like gynaecologists, bone density scans and womb ultrasounds was dependent on where you live.[6] And as I write, there are ongoing supply problems of HRT drugs in the UK, leaving patients struggling and trawling the internet for supplies.

It's challenging for sure, but things *are* changing. As well as the mega-shift in awareness, menopause is finally a focus for policymakers and politicians, workplaces are doing more to help staff, and new technology is emerging to help track hormones or treat symptoms. In 2015, NICE published its first national guidelines on menopause, and in 2020 menopause was added to the school curriculum in England for the first time.[7,8] So with a bit of luck the next generation of women will know what's coming down the line, or what might be coming, and can prepare for it. It gives me hope that we can all stop burying our heads in the sand (I can't be the only one), do the research and be ready to represent ourselves.

When I started *Why Mums Don't Jump*, I wasn't really thinking about menopause. I wasn't really thinking about older women at all. I was too busy being shocked that pelvic floor problems could happen in your twenties and thirties. And of course it is shocking, but I think that's partly because, on some level, we *expect* to face these sorts of issues later in life or we accept them as 'old lady problems', as if being over fifty, or sixty, or seventy, means you won't mind a bit of leaking or pelvic organ dislodging. Think about it for a second. It took a message from a listener to make me consider just how wrong that is. Dr Jan Russell found out she had a prolapse when she was sixty. She wrote to me to point out that having your 'fanny fall out' at that age is still 'incredibly distressing'. It's a fair point. I invited her on to the podcast.

Jan is a coach and mentor, a grandmother, an author and, as she puts it, 'a feisty old crone'. She lives in Portugal and has one of those voices that makes you feel like everything is OK with the world: calm, warm and reassuring. When we spoke she was wearing a chunky, beaded necklace, which she took off with a smile when we realized it was responsible for the mysterious clicking sound on the microphone. She's sixty-five now, but remembers the moment she realized something was wrong. She was taking a bath, and just days away from the trip of a lifetime – a transatlantic cruise to celebrate her sixtieth birthday: 'I think I had an awareness that something was going awry, but, until that moment in the bath, I wasn't 100 per cent sure what,' she told me. 'So I was alarmed. I'd got visions of being in my glad rags and dancing on the wonderful ballroom floor on this amazing ship, really not knowing what would happen next with my pelvic organs.'

Jan said she was shocked and afraid, but she really didn't want to miss the holiday that her partner had planned so carefully, so she got her act into gear and managed to get a GP appointment. The doctor explained what had happened – that it was a prolapse and that, in her view, she would 'almost certainly' need surgery. It made Jan think back to the birth of her second child, her son, thirty years earlier. She has a vague memory of the word 'prolapse' being used, but was told very little about what it meant and, back then, there was no Dr Google to ask. She was simply advised that if she wanted to avoid an operation she should do her pelvic floor exercises, which she did, for a while. And then when things felt better, she stopped and forgot all about it. So after she had her bath moment, she did what we all do, she blamed herself: 'I was scared really, of what was happening. And I felt ashamed. I felt kind of responsible . . . what have I, or haven't I done, that has meant this has happened all these years later?'

It didn't surprise me when Jan said she blamed herself. Every woman I've ever spoken to with pelvic floor issues says the same, myself included. She wondered whether it would have happened if she'd kept up the Kegels, or maybe if she hadn't been working out, unsupervised, at the gym. She'll never know. None of us will. But I'd love to understand why we do this to ourselves. Would we feel the same if it were a broken leg or a sprained wrist? Would that feeling go away if we had a better understanding of our bodies? Or if the shame and stigma around pelvic floor problems didn't exist? If we were able to get more matter of fact about it, maybe it would take away this layer of self-contempt. There's really enough to deal with, without agonizing over the what-ifs.

Jan was not going to let this get in the way of the cruise. She decided to go ahead, and I'm pleased to report that she ended up having a fabulous time. She started up her pelvic floor training again, rested when she could during the day and, yes, she danced in the evening, ignoring her fears that everything would fall out on the ballroom floor. Then, once she got home, she got a referral to see a consultant and tried to get on with life, but it wasn't easy. In those early months she had no idea what she could or couldn't do. The Fear around lifting and moving was there, but at 5'9" and looking fit and well, she didn't feel comfortable asking people for help because she didn't want to have to explain it. It started to affect her body image and her self-esteem: 'There are all kinds of connotations, aren't there? A feeling of failure. Am I still sexual? Am I still a proper woman? And it's a taboo – you don't sit around the dinner table and somebody says, "How are you?" and you go, "Well I'm fine, but my prolapse is playing up and the organs are down a bit today".' The idea of it made us both laugh. Not yet we don't, Jan. Not yet.

By the time Jan's consultant appointment came through, she was seeing a Pilates coach who recommended a pelvic health physiotherapist. With their help she was exercising and had a better understanding of what she could do. She felt like she was making progress, but her consultant felt it wouldn't be enough and offered vaginal mesh surgery. Jan turned it down: 'I'm really pleased about that because now there is much more awareness of how incredibly problematic that can be. I'm sure it has worked for some women and, if so, that's great. I also know it can be very problematic.'

For more than twenty years, vaginal (or pelvic) mesh implants have been surgically inserted to treat incontinence and prolapse by supporting the pelvic organs and damaged tissues.[9] But they've been heavily restricted in the UK since 2018, when, as we've heard, they were linked to 'crippling, life-changing, complications' in some patients.[10] Around the world, thousands of women have complained of side effects including mesh erosion (where the mesh cuts through the internal tissues), painful sex, nerve trauma and pelvic, back and leg pain. I mentioned the Cumberlege Review earlier, and it really lays bare the extent of suffering, as well as a lack of oversight – with no proper record of how many times mesh was used or of how many women have experienced problems.[11] It's a health scandal that has had a devastating effect on lives, relationships and careers, and legal cases are ongoing in the UK, the US, Canada and Australia.

It's important to say that there are other types of surgery available and that, at least when it comes to incontinence, there are non-surgical procedures too, like nerve stimulation or bladder injections. New potential treatments are being developed as well, including stem cell therapy for injured sphincter muscles and for prolapse. So it might not always seem like it, but there *are* options and hopefully more to come. When I spoke to the consultant colorectal surgeon, Julie Cornish, about it she made it clear that trying one thing doesn't mean you can't then try something else:

> There is a lot you can do yourself: look at your diet, look at your lifestyle, look at your exercise. Physiotherapy is fantastic, but it isn't the answer to everything. If it's not better, or it's not in a good place for you, do continue to seek help. And just be aware that, as we get older, things can change again.

Jan told me that, six years on, she's in a 'management process' in terms of her symptoms. She still sees a physio-therapist, she keeps up the exercise, including the strength training, and while she's 'aware' of her pelvic floor, for now, she rarely has any issues, and she's grateful for that. I asked if she knew much about any of this when she was having her children in the eighties. Did she even know what a pelvic floor was? Was it something that anybody ever spoke about? 'Oh no,' she said, 'not at all.' She remembers having a tear after her first child, her daughter, was born, and the doctor being really embarrassed to be stitching her. 'He couldn't name anything,' she said. 'He told me I'd have to wear "bunny pads" . . . He meant sanitary towels, but he couldn't say that to this woman of twenty-seven who had just given birth, you know? So that was the era.'

There are estimated to be around 13 million women in the UK alone who are currently peri- or postmenopausal, around a third of the entire female population. Around the world, that figure is expected to reach 1.2 billion by 2030.[12] That's a huge chunk of the global population and yet we're only just starting to talk more openly about it. A survey published in 2021 by the menopause awareness organization GenM found that more than half of those questioned could name just three out of the dozens of symptoms associated with menopause; two-thirds said they were 'shocked and unprepared' when it happened; and two-fifths of women going through it said they felt 'lonely, invisible, irrelevant or dispensable'.[13] Generation after generation has been walking into menopause with no clue what's happening – overlooked and underprepared for whatever symptoms turn up, just like we've been walking into pelvic floor problems after childbirth with zero knowledge of what that might mean. And it doesn't matter what age you are, the impact is real. 'We still have feelings, and thoughts about things, and anticipation of futures, you know?' Jan told me. 'And I think there's such a need for women to be able to claim visibility and empowerment at any age. We are here, and we have these bodily functions, and they shouldn't be secrets or things to be ashamed of.'

A listener in California wrote to me recently. She told me

she was fifty-nine years old and had never heard of prolapse until she was diagnosed a month earlier. 'I have seen my gynaecologist every year since I was a teenager,' she said, 'and she *never* told me this could happen.' She told me she was planning a 'vagina tea party' for her cousins, her daughters, their friends and 'basically anyone who owns a vagina'. I have no idea what that will look like, but it put a huge smile on my face. I'm imagining a garden party with cups and saucers, pastel-coloured bunting and vulva-themed cupcakes, obviously with a large slice of pelvic floor chat on the side. If I didn't live 3000 miles away, I would be there like a shot. That's the world I'd like to live in. I don't mean the tea party bit, as good as it sounds, but one where we can just be open about our gynaecological dramas, where we are taught about our bodies and taught to fight for our bodies, where we can all head towards our 'feisty old crone'.

'Be a feisty young woman,' said Jan. 'Really if we stop long enough, we do know our bodies. So fight for your body. Put your feistiness into it. You are worth looking after.'

Menopause

- The average age for menopause is fifty-one, a single day in your life that marks twelve months since your last period.
- Perimenopause is the transition to menopause and can begin several years earlier.
- Hormone changes can lead to a vast array of potential symptoms, including joint aches, irregular periods, reduced sex drive, mood changes, hot flushes and pelvic floor problems.
- Treatments include diet and lifestyle changes – eating well, sleeping well, exercising and managing stress. For some women, hormone replacement therapy (HRT) can help.
- Don't put up with not feeling well! Seek advice from a medical professional.

CHAPTER 11

POP CLUB!

(FIND YOUR PEOPLE)

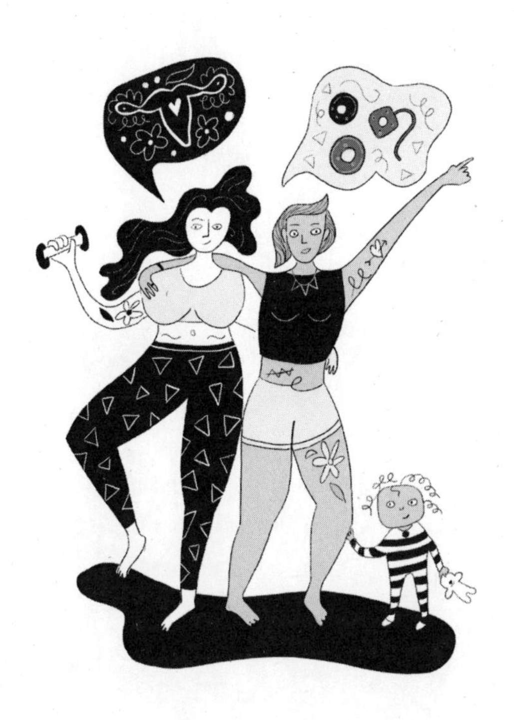

It's not every day you walk into a coffee shop to discuss your vagina with complete strangers. Or at least it wasn't when I arranged to do just that in January 2019. It was a few months after I started on Instagram – more than a year before I launched the podcast – and a message popped up from a woman in Australia. She had a friend in Manchester with a prolapse, why didn't we meet for a coffee? That would obviously be a really weird thing to do. But then again, what did I have to lose?

I arrived at the cafe with my then three-year-old son to meet Skye (not her real name, but a pseudonym rather hilariously inspired by the Australian soap opera, *Home and Away*) and her friend, Jess (also not her real name but nothing to do with nineties television). Jess had a prolapse too, and both brought their toddlers along, so it was shaping up to be quite the party. And, as bizarre as it sounds, it was brilliant. The kids happily annihilated a toy kitchen while the three of us jumped straight in, discussing our knackered nethers in depth, over tea and cake. At one point, Jess's husband made a brief appearance, as if the gathering wasn't strange enough already. And that was the inaugural meeting of our little group of pelvic organ prolapse mums, or 'POP Club!' as we decided to call it, because every good WhatsApp group needs a catchy title.

It took months, and an amount of gin, but I eventually convinced my new friends to come up with their stage names and share their experiences on the podcast. And they did it beautifully. It was in the middle of lockdown, so we were on a video call. There were missing headphones and technical glitches, but when we managed to get past all of that and start recording, Jess recalled how she first met Skye. It was at a baby group a few weeks after the birth. She'd had a rough time – an induction and a forceps delivery, which she described as traumatizing, then a stitches infection and the prolapse. She remembered the effort it took to get out of the house, worrying about where she would park, how she would get the pram out of the car, how far she would have to walk and whether there would be any stairs. Her prolapse was on her mind 24/7 and heading out was the last thing she felt like doing, but she had promised a friend she'd be there. 'I remember dragging myself out even though I just wanted to wail at home, and looking around thinking everyone's having the perfect time. I remember seeing Skye and thinking she looks really happy, with her perfect vagina.' We all laughed at this. Little did she know.

Skye remembered, too, how the two of them were sitting around chatting, probably about the storm that is new motherhood, when Jess suddenly announced her prolapse. 'It was such a breath of fresh air,' she said, 'because nobody had ever mentioned it to me before.' Skye told us she'd been 'suffering in silence', unable to talk about it, even with her closest friends, 'so for somebody to come out and say it in front of me, and to be able to relate to that was amazing, and still is to be honest.'

Skye was pretty poorly after her son was born. Like Jess, she had a forceps delivery, then she had sepsis, and she wore a catheter for five weeks. It was when that was removed that she realized things weren't healing as they should. She went to the GP and was told that everything was fine, nothing was wrong. But when weeks passed and things still didn't feel right, she returned to the doctor and asked her to take another look. 'She said, "Oh yeah, you do have a prolapse actually." And I was like, "Oh brilliant."' Skye was in pain too. She saw a private physiotherapist and discovered that, as well as the prolapse, she had a hypertonic pelvic floor (the tight one). The muscles weren't coordinating or cooperating: 'All the time I thought I was relaxing, I was just tensing in a weird way. I had no idea what was going on down there. Everything was just not as it should be. But the physio really helped, and then eventually I got to see a consultant at the hospital.'

A year and a half after the birth of her son, and not long before we all met in the cafe, Skye had surgery for her prolapse. It was a posterior repair of the back wall of the vagina. She says she went into it knowing that it wasn't going to fix everything, but it did help with some things, like making bowel movements less difficult. She later found out that some of the pain she'd been experiencing since the birth was related to nerve damage. Like Chantelle in Chapter 5, she had pudendal neuralgia, where the main nerve in the pelvis is harmed or irritated.[1] It can cause long-term pain in any part of the pelvic area, and childbirth is one of a number of possible causes. There are no specific tests for it, so it's difficult to diagnose, and it's not known how many people are affected.[2] Treatments include lifestyle changes and physiotherapy, as well as painkilling injections, surgery and nerve stimulation, but not all of these are widely available.[3]

Pain is still an issue for Skye, although she thinks it's slowly improving, or that she's managing it better. She told us she does the exercises her physio gave her every day and we teased her about being a model patient. She said her injuries don't stop her living the life she wants to live, whether it's running, or climbing mountains, or just being daft with her little boy. 'I was still dancing around the room to eighties power ballads tonight carrying my toddler, so it can't be that bad, can it?' she joked. 'I mean, I deal with it.' She explained that she was referred back to the hospital for the pain, but it was cancelled because of Covid. At which point, a concerned Jess told her, in no uncertain terms, 'That needs looking at. You need to follow it up.'

In her own, inimitable way, Jess told us how *she* became aware of her pelvic floor issues when her son was just eight days old. 'I don't really like this story,' she said. She had walked a mile or so to a restaurant and back, and everything felt heavy and uncomfortable. Then she wrestled with a heavy car seat on the way to a GP appointment for her wound infection. 'That was probably the icing on the cake,' she said. 'I don't really remember much after that. It was a year and a half of misery. It sounds really depressing, but it was. There were joyous times in it as well, but I was just really worried about everything: "I won't be the mum I want to be, I want to play rounders, I want to run, I want to chase, I want to lift, I want to run down the street with my son when he's older." There were a lot of times when I just got myself through with some box sets on Netflix.'

Jess told us she's feeling better these days, and then she entertained us with a funny story about being fitted for a pessary. I can't do it justice here (you'll have to listen to the podcast), but the key point is that it helped and, although she still has symptoms of discomfort and constipation, she thinks she's 'coming to terms with it'. She tries to worry a bit less, to get past The Fear. She confessed that she used to think Skye was 'crazy' for riding a bike, but that she rode one recently, for the first time since her son's birth, two-and-a-half years earlier. And she loved it. 'My son was on the back and I was a bit teary,' she told us. 'It was an emotional moment because this was the mum that I always wanted to be, *this* person.'

We talked about how poorly prepared we were for the realities of postpartum recovery, with wholly unrealistic expectations of what we should or shouldn't be able to do. 'I had forceps,' Jess said, 'and I was out of hospital within a day, with no real advice.' She pointed to social media too, and the pressure that still exists for mums to 'snap back' after birth, wondering if she overdid the walking or the lifting. There's the self-blame again. And although it does feel sometimes like that narrative is changing, it's still true that for every article or post that endorses body positivity, there's another that celebrates shedding the baby weight or a swift return to the gym. Celebrities are pictured 'flaunting' their postpartum weight loss or 'showing off' their return to a pre-pregnancy figure. It's damaging in so many ways. And it's another reason why we need to share real stories, with all their wobbly bits: the good, the bad, the ugly and the cringe.

Jess smiled as she described how she started to make it her quest to try to find other mums with pelvic floor troubles, casually bringing it up whenever she got the chance, in the park, with friends from her antenatal group, at the Trafford Centre (there is something about that fountain). She said it was her way of coping. Skye's at it now too. As I write, she's on holiday in Majorca where she told us she's been discussing vaginas with a woman she met at the hotel, who also has a prolapse. It's catching (the talking, not the prolapse), like dominoes falling. When I opened up about my own experience, other mums started seeking me out at the school gate, at work or in the pub to share their stories; one ran towards me across a crowded bar shouting 'I have a prolapse!', and gave me a big hug, which was surprising, but also wonderful.

The podcast has had a similar effect: a chain reaction of people around the world listening to other women's stories and feeling inspired to share their own – quietly with partners or friends, noisily in national newspapers, or discreetly in a message to me. 'Thank you for the hope,' they say. 'It's so comforting to know I'm not alone.' They tell me the podcast has made them cry 'in a good way' and that they have 'never felt so seen'. And then there was this classic: 'Buggered fannies really do love company.'

After the POP Club! episode went out, people kept asking where they could find their local branch, and I kept having to explain that it wasn't an official sort of set-up. But then an amazing thing happened. Women from all over the UK started to connect through my Instagram account – from Sheffield to Bristol, York to South Wales, Newcastle to London and as far away as Canada, the US and New Zealand – meeting for walks, and coffees, and drinks. One woman got in touch to say the two-member Ayrshire contingent had gone rollerblading around a fancy Scottish golf course. 'I think both of us were so over being coy,' she wrote. 'Let's just say the golfers got an education that evening.' It's an image that I will always treasure.

It's such a powerful thing to realize that you're not on your own with your pelvic floor problems – that the struggle you thought was unique to you is being experienced by others at exactly the same time, and often in the same way: the shock, the grief, the self-blame, the anger and the questioning. It sounds obvious. In this age of endless information, you'd think you would know that this was the case, but because it's all so hidden, it's like someone is reading your mind when they voice all the same thoughts and fears – and it's validating. It's not just you. You didn't do anything wrong. You are not failing.

It's empowering too. Meeting Skye and Jess, and *all* of the brave and brilliant women I've spoken to, has made a profound difference to how I view my own pelvic floor dysfunction. Somehow, hearing their experiences has helped me to come to terms with mine. It has watered down the shame and embarrassment, given me a route back to exercise and encouraged me to try pessaries again – real-world changes that have helped me to become more like the mum I imagined I would be all those years ago. And it's not just me. I know it's had a similar effect on others. Women who have pushed for pelvic health physio or pessaries after years of suffering, who have had conversations with their doctor about treatment or their boss about managing at work, who have signed up for pelvic floor and core workout programmes, or who have found determination and comfort through dark times. I've worked in radio for twenty years, so I thought I understood the power of sharing stories, but I see now that I underestimated the lasting impact it can have. 'BTW, just found your podcast on Spotify,' wrote one woman, 'and it has changed my life.'

Towards the end of that first season, I had a message from a woman in London. Her name was Cat Pearson and she was a new mum who'd been struggling with prolapse and pelvic pain. She came across a link to the podcast in a London parents' group and it had helped her out of a bad head space: 'I've been so frustrated about the lack of good information out there,' she wrote, 'and while I've just sat around on my (very painful) arse and done nothing about it, I'm so happy that you have!' Cat told me she was a designer, and she volunteered her services to help get the message out there, an offer which I obviously grabbed with both hands.

I thought Cat might be able to improve on my home-made logo, but, as it happened, she had much bigger ideas. She did design a new logo, and then also created an entire brand identity that was beyond my wildest dreams: noisy, unapologetic and proud, with a series of beautiful, line-drawn illustrations which celebrate the wonky bodies we can sometimes be left with – you will have seen them throughout this book. We worked together over Zoom during the Covid pandemic and, as a listener, she understood exactly what the podcast was about, often articulating it far better than I ever could. After months of using my endlessly patient husband as a sounding board, it was reaffirming to have someone else who really 'got it'.

Cat later told me that when she first heard the podcast it made her laugh and cry, and it also made her realize how angry she felt. 'Angry, because I'd just gone back to work after maternity leave, and I was telling people I had a sore back because their faces looked so awkward when I tried to explain the full details.' She was fed up with the shame and secrecy, fed up with squirming. She wanted to flip the switch, and she did. By the time season two launched, she'd gone from hiding her condition to blogging about it, and roping me in for a shared presentation at a work event. I told you it was catching.

A few years ago, sitting on the bedroom floor in my sorry state, I felt like my body had changed so fundamentally that I would never find myself again. I was thirty-six and over the hill. I had peaked and missed it. But then something magical happened. We found ways to say the unsayable, and the sky didn't fall in. And now we're part of something that feels bigger, where women's health and pelvic floors are starting to emerge from the shadows, on social media and on podcasts, but also on TV programmes and in newspapers, as well as in government policy documents and in the national health guidelines. I recently read that pelvic health was a 'top fitness trend' which is an odd way to describe something so fundamental to our well-being, but I'll take it. I'll celebrate anything that chips away at the stubborn taboo that leaves so many people suffering in silence.

I am a work in progress. Sometimes I do all the things that help me to feel better: eating well, pelvic floor exercises, running, Pilates, yoga. Then sometimes life gets in the way, and I do none of it for ages. Sometimes my prolapse feels fine; sometimes it doesn't. I'm never really sure if it's because of something I have or haven't done, if it's hormonal, or I'm just more conscious of it. Maybe it will get worse over time; maybe it won't. But the big difference is that it doesn't consume me in the way it once did. It's not on my mind all the time, dictating what I do, how I move and how I feel.

I don't have all the answers, but I do have hope. Hope,

that by sharing these stories, others can get there sooner than I did; skipping the shock, shame and blame, and going straight to the part where there's rehabilitation and support; where we can all learn to reclaim our lives in full technicolour glory. Hope, that by amplifying these voices, it will make it easier for others to speak out, and trigger the change that we deserve for ourselves, our friends, our colleagues and our children. Because, when we come together, we are stronger and much harder to ignore.

Community

- Meeting other women with pelvic floor problems, online and in person, has really helped me to come to terms with my own experience.
- Find *your* people! You'll be amazed by the support you will find and can offer to others.
- We all have good days and bad, so try not to beat yourself up if you're not on top of everything.
- Please don't be afraid or embarrassed to seek professional help.
- And remember, you are not alone, and there is *always* hope.

Resources

As you know, I really struggled to find any decent information or support for my pelvic floor problems. The good news is that things are slowly improving. There are some excellent resources out there, once you know where to look. Below are some of the ones that I have found useful, or that have been recommended to me.

Websites

Association for Pelvic Organ Prolapse Support (APOPS)
A US-based non-profit organization which provides guidance and support to women navigating pelvic organ prolapse.
https://www.pelvicorganprolapsesupport.org/

The Birth Trauma Association
A charity that supports women who suffer birth trauma.
https://www.birthtraumaassociation.org.uk/

Bladder & Bowel Community
A support network for people affected by bladder and bowel conditions.
https://www.bladderandbowel.org/

Make Birth Better
A collective of parents and professionals working together to end suffering from birth trauma.
https://www.makebirthbetter.org/

MASIC
A charity for mothers with anal sphincter injuries in childbirth.
https://masic.org.uk/

Maternal Mental Health Alliance
A campaign to improve perinatal mental health care.
https://maternalmentalhealthalliance.org/

NHS
Easy-to-read and up-to-date information on pelvic floor problems and treatments.
https://www.nhs.uk/conditions/

PANDAS Foundation UK
Support for people coping with perinatal mental illnesses, as well as their families, friends and carers.
https://www.pandasfoundation.org.uk/

Pelvic Obstetric & Gynaecological Physiotherapy (POGP)

A professional network of physiotherapists with a professional interest in women's (and men's) health. They have some really well-written patient information booklets.
https://thepogp.co.uk/default.aspx

Pelvic Roar

A physiotherapy-led pelvic health campaign.
https://www.pelvicroar.org/

Royal College of Obstetricians & Gynaecologists (RCOG)

The professional body responsible for the development and training of people who work in obstetrics and gynaecology. They also have some good patient information leaflets about pelvic floor dysfunction.
https://www.rcog.org.uk/

Fitness websites

Holistic Core Restore

Pelvic floor and core fitness.
https://www.holisticcorerestore.com/

MUTU System

An online postnatal exercise programme.
https://mutusystem.co.uk/

POPUp

Online resources for managing pelvic organ prolapse.
https://www.popuplifting.com/

Books

Invisible Women: Exposing data bias in a world designed for men, Caroline Criado Perez (Chatto & Windus, 2019)

It's About Bloody Time. Period, Emma Barnett (HQ, 2021)

PMSL: Or how I literally pissed myself laughing and survived the last taboo to tell the tale, Luce Brett (Green Tree, 2020)

Raising the Skirt: The unsung power of the vagina, Catherine Blackledge (W&N, 2020)

Rebel Bodies: A guide to the gender health gap revolution, Sarah Graham (Bloomsbury, 2023)

Vagina: A re-education, Lynn Enright (Allen & Unwin, 2019)

Why Did No One Tell Me? How to protect, heal and nurture your body through motherhood, Emma Brockwell (Vermilion, 2021)

Your Pelvic Floor: A practical guide to solving your most intimate problems, Kim Vopni (Watkins Publishing, 2021)

Documentary

Sophie Power: The Journey from Pregnancy to Performance, https://youtu.be/9QcbaUux5oI (Hoka, 2021)

Apps

Couch to 5K
A running app for beginners. If you have pelvic floor problems, take advice from a health professional first.

https://www.nhs.uk/live-well/exercise/running-and-aerobic-exercises/get-running-with-couch-to-5k/

Squeezy

An NHS app which will remind you to do your pelvic floor exercises by sending a notification to your phone. It's very persistent so it's fairly effective! It also has a directory of pelvic health physios so you can find one near you.
https://squeezyapp.com/

Instagram

@clarebournephysio: Clare Bourne, pelvic health physiotherapist

@gusset_grippers: Fellow of the Chartered Society of Physiotherapy and comedian

@gynaegirl: Tiffany Sequeira, pelvic health physiotherapist

@jillybondphysio: Jilly Bond, pelvic health physiotherapist

@physiomumuk: Emma Brockwell, pelvic health physiotherapist

@tears_from_tearing: Chantelle Sandham, birth-injured mum

@the.vagina.whisperer: Dr Sara Reardon, pelvic floor physical therapist

@whymumsdontjump: Helen Ledwick, mum with a prolapse. And a podcast. And a book.

Podcasts

At Your Cervix
A podcast dedicated to pelvic and women's health issues such as incontinence, pelvic pain or sexual dysfunction, hosted by physiotherapists Emma Brockwell and Gráinne Donnelly.

Bits of Me
A podcast about women's bodies, all the things we should know about them and all the stories behind them, hosted by journalist Linnea Dunne.

Mother Bodies
A podcast about health after birth – and why it matters, hosted by journalist Rosie Taylor.

The Lowdown with Bravemumma
A podcast supporting women with pelvic organ prolapse, hosted by Stephanie Thompson.

The Pelvic Health Podcast
A podcast for professionals, as well as the general public, on all things related to pelvic health, hosted by physical therapist Lori Forner.

Why Mums Don't Jump
A kick-ass podcast about lumps and leaks after childbirth, hosted by me, Helen Ledwick.

References

INTRODUCTION

1 Lawrence, J. M., Lukacz, E. S., Nager, C. W., Hsu, J. W. Y., & Luber, K. M. (2008). Prevalence and co-occurrence of pelvic floor disorders in community-dwelling women. *Obstetrics & Gynecology*, 111(3), 678–85.

2 Mazi, B., Kaddour, O., & Al-Badr, A. (2019). Depression symptoms in women with pelvic floor dysfunction: A case-control study. *International Journal of Women's Health*, 11, 143.

3 The Independent Medicines and Medical Devices Safety Review (2020). *First Do No Harm*. Retrieved from https://www.immdsreview.org.uk/downloads/IMMDSReview_Web.pdf.

4 Department of Health & Social Care (6 Mar. 2021). Government launches call for evidence to improve health and wellbeing of women in England. Retrieved from https://www.gov.uk/government/consultations/womens-health-strategy-call-for-evidence/womens-health-strategy-call-for-evidence.

5 Graham, S. (13 May 2022). British women are still clueless

about their bodies because reproductive education is not cutting through. *i*. Retrieved from https://inews.co.uk/opinion/british-women-are-still-clueless-about-their-bodies-because-reproductive-education-is-not-cutting-through-1625824.

6 Lawrence, J. M., Lukacz, E. S., Nager, C. W., Hsu, J. W. Y., & Luber, K. M. (2008). Prevalence and co-occurrence of pelvic floor disorders in community-dwelling women. *Obstetrics & Gynecology*, 111(3), 678–85.

CHAPTER 1: MY STORY

1 National Institute for Health and Care Excellence (24 Jun. 2019). Urinary incontinence and pelvic organ prolapse in women: Management. Retrieved from https://www.nice.org.uk/guidance/ng123/chapter/Context.

2 Royal College of Obstetricians & Gynaecologists (n.d.). Third- and fourth-degree tears (OASI). Retrieved from https://www.rcog.org.uk/for-the-public/perineal-tears-and-episiotomies-in-childbirth/third-and-fourth-degree-tears-oasi/.

3 Huber, M., Malers, E., & Tunón, K. (2021). Pelvic floor dysfunction one year after first childbirth in relation to perineal tear severity. *Scientific Reports*, 11(1), 12560.

4 Sideris, M., McCaughey, T., Hanrahan, J. G., Arroyo-Manzano, D., Zamora, J., Jha, S., et al (2020). Risk of obstetric anal sphincter injuries (OASIS) and anal incontinence: A meta-analysis. *European Journal of Obstetrics & Gynecology and Reproductive Biology*, 252, 303–12.

5 Royal College of Obstetricians & Gynaecologists (29 Oct. 2019). Care of a third- or fourth-degree tear that occurred during childbirth (also known as obstetric anal sphincter injury OASI). Retrieved from https://www.rcog.org.uk/for-the-public/browse-all-patient-information-leaflets/care-of-a-third-or-

fourth-degree-tear-that-occurred-during-childbirth-also-known-as-obstetric-anal-sphincter-injury-oasi/.

6 MASIC (Jul. 2021). Breaking the taboo: The impact of severe maternal birth injuries on the mother–baby bond. Retrieved from https://masic.org.uk/wp-content/uploads/2021/05/MASIC-survey-V4.pdf.

7 NHS (23 Dec. 2019). Risks: Hip replacement. Retrieved from https://www.nhs.uk/conditions/hip-replacement/risks/#:~:text=Hip%20replacement%20surgery%20is%20done,an%20infection%20may%20still%20happen.

8 NHS (7 May 2020). Treatment: Varicose veins. Retrieved from https://www.nhs.uk/conditions/varicose-veins/treatment/.

9 Sideris, M., McCaughey, T., Hanrahan, J. G., Arroyo-Manzano, D., Zamora, J., Jha, S., et al (2020). Risk of obstetric anal sphincter injuries (OASIS) and anal incontinence: A meta-analysis. *European Journal of Obstetrics & Gynecology and Reproductive Biology*, 252, 303–12.

10 Powell, W. (n.d.). #IWishIKnew. MUTU System. Retrieved from https://mutusystem.com/en-uk/mutu-pregnancy/i-wish-i-knew/.

CHAPTER 2: AINSLEY (THE DOCTOR WILL SEE YOU NOW)

1 International Continence Society (2022). Urinary incontinence symptoms. Retrieved from https://www.ics.org/glossary/symptom/urinaryincontinence.

2 Buckley, B. S., & Lapitan, M. C. M. (2010). Prevalence of urinary incontinence in men, women, and children – current evidence: Findings of the Fourth International Consultation on Incontinence. *Urology*, 76(2), 265–70.

3 Ibid.

4 National Institute for Health and Care Excellence (Oct. 2019). What are the causes and contributing factors for urinary

incontinence? Retrieved from https://cks.nice.org.uk/topics/incontinence-urinary-in-women/background-information/causes-contributing-factors/.

5 Gümüşsoy, S., Kavlak, O., & Dönmez, S. (2019). Investigation of body image, self-esteem, and quality of life in women with urinary incontinence. *International Journal of Nursing Practice*, 25(5), e12762.

6 Dumoulin, C., Cacciari, L. P., & Hay-Smith, E. J. C. (2018). Pelvic floor muscle training versus no treatment, or inactive control treatments, for urinary incontinence in women. *Cochrane Database of Systematic Reviews*, (10).

7 HM Government (Sep. 2021). Build back better: Our plan for health and social care. Retrieved from https://assets.publishing.service.gov.uk/government/uploads/system/uploads/attachment_data/file/1015736/Build_Back_Better-_Our_Plan_for_Health_and_Social_Care.pdf.

8 Royal College of Obstetricians & Gynaecologists (4 Apr. 2022). More than half a million women face prolonged waits for gynaecology care. Retrieved from https://www.rcog.org.uk/news/more-than-half-a-million-women-face-prolonged-waits-for-gynaecology-care/.

9 Ibid.

10 Kelly, H. (29 Sep. 2021). Mother of all injustices! Mums injured in labour are denied health insurance payouts yet their husbands are covered for football injuries on same policy. *Daily Mail*. Retrieved from https://www.thisismoney.co.uk/money/bills/article-10037489/Mums-criticise-health-insurers-denying-birth-claims.html.

11 The Independent Medicines and Medical Devices Safety Review (2020). *First Do No Harm*. Retrieved from https://www.immdsreview.org.uk/downloads/IMMDSReview_Web.pdf.

12 National Institute for Health and Care Excellence (9 Dec. 2021). Pelvic floor dysfunction: Prevention and non-surgical management. Retrieved from https://www.nice.org.uk/guidance/ng210/resources/pelvic-floor-dysfunction-prevention-and-nonsurgical-management-pdf-66143768482501.

13 NHS (n.d.). Maternity and neonatal services. Retrieved from https://www.longtermplan.nhs.uk/online-version/chapter-3-further-progress-on-care-quality-and-outcomes/a-strong-start-in-life-for-children-and-young-people/maternity-and-neonatal-services/.

14 NHS England (13 Jun. 2021). NHS pelvic health clinics to help tens of thousands of women across the country. Retrieved from https://www.england.nhs.uk/2021/06/nhs-pelvic-health-clinics-to-help-tens-of-thousands-women-across-the-country/.

15 National Institute for Health and Care Excellence (9 Dec. 2021). Pelvic floor dysfunction: Prevention and non-surgical management. Overview. Retrieved from https://www.nice.org.uk/guidance/ng210.

16 National Institute for Health and Care Excellence (n.d.). Guidelines scope: Pelvic floor dysfunction: prevention and non-surgical management. Retrieved from https://www.nice.org.uk/guidance/ng210/documents/final-scope.

17 Abhyankar, P., Wilkinson, J., Berry, K., Wane, S., Uny, I., Aitchison, P., et al (2020). Implementing pelvic floor muscle training for women with pelvic organ prolapse: A realist evaluation of different delivery models. *BMC Health Services Research*, 20(1), 1–16.

18 National Institute for Health and Care Excellence (9 Dec. 2021). Pelvic floor dysfunction: Prevention and non-surgical management. Rationale and impact. Retrieved from https://www.nice.org.uk/guidance/ng210/chapter/Rationale-and-impact.

19 Horak, T. A., Guzman-Rojas, R. A., Shek, K. L. L., & Dietz, H. P. (2014). Pelvic floor trauma: Does the second baby matter? *Ultrasound in Obstetrics & Gynecology*, 44(1), 90–4.

20 Jundt, K., Scheer, I., von Bodungen, V., Krumbachner, F., Friese, K., & Peschers, U. M. (2010). What harm does a second delivery to the pelvic floor? *European Journal of Medical Research*, 15(8), 362–6.

21 International Continence Society (n.d.). Urinary incontinence symptoms. Retrieved from https://www.ics.org/glossary/symptom/urinaryincontinence.

22 Buckley, B. S., & Lapitan, M. C. M. (2010). Prevalence of urinary incontinence in men, women, and children – current evidence: Findings of the Fourth International Consultation on Incontinence. *Urology*, 76(2), 265–70.

23 Dumoulin, C., Cacciari, L. P., & Hay-Smith, E. J. C. (2018). Pelvic floor muscle training versus no treatment, or inactive control treatments, for urinary incontinence in women. *Cochrane Database of Systematic Reviews*, (10).

CHAPTER 3: PEACE (EDUCATION, EDUCATION, EDUCATION)

1 El-Hamamsy, D., Parmar, C., Shoop-Worrall, S., & Reid, F. M. (2022). Public understanding of female genital anatomy and pelvic organ prolapse (POP); A questionnaire-based pilot study. *International Urogynecology Journal*, 33(2), 309–18.

2 Geddes, L. (30 May 2021). Most Britons cannot name all parts of the vulva, survey reveals. *Guardian*. Retrieved from https://www.theguardian.com/lifeandstyle/2021/may/30/most-britons-cannot-name-parts-vulva-survey.

3 Graham, S. (13 May 2022). British women are still clueless about their bodies because reproductive education is not cutting through. *i*. Retrieved from https://inews.co.uk/opinion/british-women-are-still-clueless-about-their-bodies-

because-reproductive-education-is-not-cutting-through-1625824.

4 National Institute for Health and Care Excellence (9 Dec. 2021). Pelvic floor dysfunction: Prevention and non-surgical management. Overview. Retrieved from https://www.nice.org.uk/guidance/ng210/chapter/Recommendations#preventing-pelvic-floor-dysfunction.

5 National Institute for Health and Care Excellence (9 Dec. 2021). Pelvic floor dysfunction: Prevention and non-surgical management. Recommendations. Retrieved from https://www.nice.org.uk/guidance/ng210/chapter/Recommendations.

6 Hebert-Beirne, J. M., O'Conor, R., Ihm, J. D., Parlier, M. K., Lavender, M. D., & Brubaker, L. (2017). A pelvic health curriculum in school settings: The effect on adolescent females' knowledge. *Journal of Pediatric and Adolescent Gynecology*, 30(2), 188–92.

7 Graham, S. (13 May 2022). British women are still clueless about their bodies because reproductive education is not cutting through. *i*. Retrieved from https://inews.co.uk/opinion/british-women-are-still-clueless-about-their-bodies-because-reproductive-education-is-not-cutting-through-1625824.

8 El-Hamamsy, D., Parmar, C., Shoop-Worrall, S., & Reid, F. M. (2022). Public understanding of female genital anatomy and pelvic organ prolapse (POP); A questionnaire-based pilot study. *International Urogynecology Journal*, 33(2), 309–18.

9 National Institute for Health and Care Excellence (9 Dec. 2021). Pelvic floor dysfunction: Prevention and non-surgical management. Recommendations. Retrieved from https://www.nice.org.uk/guidance/ng210/chapter/Recommendations.

References

CHAPTER 4: SARA (THE HEAD GAME)

1. Mazi, B., Kaddour, O., & Al-Badr, A. (2019). Depression symptoms in women with pelvic floor dysfunction: A case-control study. *International Journal of Women's Health*, 11, 143.
2. Gümüşsoy, S., Kavlak, O., & Dönmez, S. (2019). Investigation of body image, self-esteem, and quality of life in women with urinary incontinence. *International Journal of Nursing Practice*, 25(5), e12762.
3. Zielinski, R., Miller, J., Low, L. K., Sampselle, C., & DeLancey, J. O. (2012). The relationship between pelvic organ prolapse, genital body image, and sexual health. *Neurourology and Urodynamics*, 31(7), 1145–8.
4. Memon, H. U., & Handa, V. L. (2013). Vaginal childbirth and pelvic floor disorders. *Women's Health*, 9(3), 265–77.
5. The Birth Trauma Association (n.d.). Retrieved from https://www.birthtraumaassociation.org.uk/.
6. Chen, Q., Li, W., Xiong, J., & Zheng, X. (2022). Prevalence and risk factors associated with postpartum depression during the COVID-19 pandemic: A literature review and meta-analysis. *International Journal of Environmental Research and Public Health*, 19(4), 2219.
7. Fultz, N., Girts, T., Kinchen, K., Nygaard, I., Pohl, G., & Sternfeld, B. (2005). Prevalence, management and impact of urinary incontinence in the workplace. *Occupational Medicine*, 55(7), 552–7.
8. Mazi, B., Kaddour, O., & Al-Badr, A. (2019). Depression symptoms in women with pelvic floor dysfunction: A case-control study. *International Journal of Women's Health*, 11, 143.

CHAPTER 5: CHANTELLE (THE TABOO)

1 Gross, R. E. (21 Sep. 2021). Taking the 'shame part' out of female anatomy. *New York Times*. Retrieved from https://www.nytimes.com/2021/09/21/science/pudendum-women-anatomy.html.

2 ISAPS (n.d.). ISAPS international survey on aesthetic/cosmetic procedures performed in 2019. Retrieved from https://www.isaps.org/wp-content/uploads/2020/12/Global-Survey-2019.pdf.

3 NHS (25 Jan. 2021). Vaginal discharge. Retrieved from https://www.nhs.uk/conditions/vaginal-discharge/.

4 Woodley, S. J., Lawrenson, P., Boyle, R., Cody, J. D., Mørkved, S., Kernohan, A., & Hay-Smith, E. J. C. (2020). Pelvic floor muscle training for preventing and treating urinary and faecal incontinence in antenatal and postnatal women. *Cochrane Database of Systematic Reviews*, (5).

5 Sharma, A., Yuan, L., Marshall, R. J., Merrie, A. E. H., & Bissett, I. P. (2016). Systematic review of the prevalence of faecal incontinence. *Journal of British Surgery*, 103(12), 1589–97.

6 Brown, H. W., Wexner, S. D., & Lukacz, E. S. (2013). Factors associated with care seeking among women with accidental bowel leakage. *Female Pelvic Medicine & Reconstructive Surgery*, 19(2), 66–71.

7 Handa, V. L., Cundiff, G., Chang, H. H., & Helzlsouer, K. J. (2008). Female sexual function and pelvic floor disorders. *Obstetrics and Gynecology*, 111(5), 1045.

8 Woodley, S. J., Lawrenson, P., Boyle, R., Cody, J. D., Mørkved, S., Kernohan, A., & Hay-Smith, E. J. C. (2020). Pelvic floor muscle training for preventing and treating urinary and faecal incontinence in antenatal and postnatal women. *Cochrane Database of Systematic Reviews*, (5).

9 Sideris, M., McCaughey, T., Hanrahan, J. G., Arroyo-Manzano, D., Zamora, J., Jha, S., et al (2020). Risk of obstetric anal sphincter injuries (OASIS) and anal incontinence: A meta-analysis. *European Journal of Obstetrics & Gynecology and Reproductive Biology*, 252, 303–12.

CHAPTER 6: SOPHIE (FINDING FITNESS)

1 Bø, K., & Nygaard, I. E. (2020). Is physical activity good or bad for the female pelvic floor? A narrative review. *Sports Medicine*, 50(3), 471–84.
2 HOKA (11 Mar. 2021). *Sophie Power: The Journey from Pregnancy to Performance* [video]. Retrieved from https://youtu.be/9QcbaUux5oI.
3 Goom, T., Donnelly, G., & Brockwell, E. (2019). Returning to running postnatal – guidelines for medical, health and fitness professionals managing this population. *Absolute Physio*.
4 National Institute for Health and Care Excellence (Dec. 2021). Pelvic floor dysfunction: Prevention and non-surgical management. Retrieved from https://www.nice.org.uk/guidance/ng210/evidence/l-physical-activity-for-the-management-of-symptoms-pdf-392138593239.
5 World Health Organization (26 Nov. 2020). Physical activity. Retrieved from https://www.who.int/news-room/fact-sheets/detail/physical-activity#:~:text=Worldwide%2C%20around%201%20in%203,physical%20activity%20to%20stay%20healthy.&text=Insufficient%20activity%20increased%20by%205,countries%20between%202001%20and%202016.
6 Hesketh, K. R., Goodfellow, L., Ekelund, U., McMinn, A. M., Godfrey, K. M., Inskip, H. M., et al (2014). Activity levels in mothers and their preschool children. *Pediatrics*, 133(4), e973–80.
7 Dakic, J. G., Cook, J., Hay-Smith, J., Lin, K. Y., Ekegren, C., & Frawley, H. C. (2022). Pelvic floor symptoms are an overlooked

barrier to exercise participation: A cross-sectional online survey of 4556 women who are symptomatic. *Physical Therapy*, 102(3), pzab284.

CHAPTER 7: RACHEL (YOU DON'T JUST PUT UP WITH IT)

1 Gervais, R. (20 Oct. 2014). It's better to create something . . . [Tweet.] Twitter. Retrieved from https://twitter.com/rickygervais/status/524131334923780096?s=20&t=x9k62Lxob1kGV2EvYgea1w.
2 Coherent Market Insights (20 Jul. 2021). Global adult incontinence products market to surpass US$ 15,845.1 million by 2027, says Coherent Market Insights (CMI). GlobeNewswire. Retrieved from https://www.globenewswire.com/en/news-release/2021/07/20/2265803/0/en/Global-Adult-Incontinence-Products-Market-to-surpass-US-15-845-1-million-by-2027-Says-Coherent-Market-Insights-CMI.html.
3 NHS England (Jun. 2018). Excellence in continence care. Retrieved from https://www.england.nhs.uk/wp-content/uploads/2018/07/excellence-in-continence-care.pdf.
4 Royal College of Nursing (Sep. 2019). RCN bulletin 379. Retrieved from https://www.rcn.org.uk/news-and-events/rcn-magazines/bul-379.
5 BBC News (5 Aug. 2019). TENA advert criticised for 'normalising' incontinence after childbirth. Retrieved from https://www.bbc.co.uk/news/uk-49235784.
6 Naidu, R., & Ando R. (22 Oct. 2019). Diaper rush: Conquering a $9 billion market no one wants to talk about. Reuters. Retrieved from https://www.reuters.com/article/us-diapers-adults-focus-idUSKBN1X10G0.
7 Natracare (n.d.). Study reveals 73% of people assume only elderly women suffer with urinary incontinence. Retrieved from https://www.natracare.com/blog/study-reveals-assumption-

only-elderly-women-suffer-urinary-incontinence/.
8 Jarbøl, D. E., Haastrup, P. F., Rasmussen, S., Søndergaaard, J., & Balasubramaniam, K. (2021). Women's barriers for contacting their general practitioner when bothered by urinary incontinence: A population-based cross-sectional study. *BMC Urology*, 21(1), 1–10.
9 Abhyankar, P., Uny, I., Semple, K., Wane, S., Hagen, S., Wilkinson, J., et al (2019). Women's experiences of receiving care for pelvic organ prolapse: A qualitative study. *BMC Women's Health*, 19(1), 1–12.

CHAPTER 8: EMMA (MIND THE GAP)

1 Department of Health & Social Care (6 Mar. 2021). Government launches call for evidence to improve health and wellbeing of women in England. Retrieved from https://www.gov.uk/government/consultations/womens-health-strategy-call-for-evidence/womens-health-strategy-call-for-evidence.
2 Winchester, N. (1 Jul. 2021). Women's health outcomes: Is there a gender gap? House of Lords Library. Retrieved from https://lordslibrary.parliament.uk/womens-health-outcomes-is-there-a-gender-gap/.
3 Department of Health & Social Care (19 Dec. 2018). The women's mental health taskforce. Retrieved from https://assets.publishing.service.gov.uk/government/uploads/system/uploads/attachment_data/file/765821/The_Womens_Mental_Health_Taskforce_-_final_report1.pdf.
4 Cooper, C., Lodwick, R., Walters, K., Raine, R., Manthorpe, J., Iliffe, S., & Petersen, I. (2017). Inequalities in receipt of mental and physical healthcare in people with dementia in the UK. *Age and Ageing*, 46(3), 393–400.
5 University of Leeds (16 Jul. 2018). Women more at risk of dying after a heart attack. Retrieved from https://www.leeds.ac.uk/

news/article/4269/women_more_at_risk_of_dying_after_a_heart_attack.

6 Chen, E. H., Shofer, F. S., Dean, A. J., Hollander, J. E., Baxt, W. G., Robey, J. L., et al (2008). Gender disparity in analgesic treatment of emergency department patients with acute abdominal pain. *Academic Emergency Medicine*, 15(5), 414–8.

7 Zhang, L., Losin, E. A. R., Ashar, Y. K., Koban, L., & Wager, T. D. (2021). Gender biases in estimation of others' pain. *The Journal of Pain*, 22(9), 1048–59.

8 News@TheU (6 Apr. 2021). Research identifies gender bias in estimation of patients' pain. University of Miami. Retrieved from https://news.miami.edu/stories/2021/04/research-identifies-gender-bias-in-estimation-of-patients-pain.html.

9 The Independent Medicines and Medical Devices Safety Review (2020). *First Do No Harm*. Retrieved from https://www.immdsreview.org.uk/downloads/IMMDSReview_Web.pdf.

10 MBRRACE-UK (2021). Saving lives, improving mothers' care. Lay summary 2021. Oxford Population Health NPEU. Retrieved from https://www.npeu.ox.ac.uk/assets/downloads/mbrrace-uk/reports/maternal-report-2021/MBRRACE-UK_Maternal_Report_2021_-_Lay_Summary_v10.pdf.

11 Office for National Statistics (25 Apr. 2022). Health state life expectancies by national deprivation deciles, England: 2018 to 2020. Retrieved from https://www.ons.gov.uk/peoplepopulationandcommunity/healthandsocialcare/healthinequalities/bulletins/healthstatelifeexpectanciesbyindexofmultipledeprivationimd/2018to2020.

12 McDermott, E., Nelson, R., & Weeks, H. (2021). The politics of LGBT+ health inequality: conclusions from a UK scoping review. *International Journal of Environmental Research and Public Health*, 18(2), 826.

13 Criado Perez, C. (2019). *Invisible Women: Exposing data bias in a world designed for men*, Chatto & Windus.
14 World Health Organization (31 Mar. 2021). Endometriosis. Retrieved from https://www.who.int/news-room/fact-sheets/detail/endometriosis#:~:text=Endometriosis%20is%20a%20disease%20where,and%20girls%20globally%20(2).
15 All Party Parliamentary Group on Endometriosis (2020). Endometriosis in the UK: Time for change. Retrieved from https://www.endometriosis-uk.org/sites/default/files/files/Endometriosis%20APPG%20Report%20Oct%202020.pdf.
16 BBC News (20 Jul. 2022). Women's health: 'I had periods that lasted for months' [video]. Retrieved from https://www.bbc.co.uk/news/av/health-62229951.
17 Department of Health & Social Care (30 Aug. 2022). Women's Health Strategy for England. Retrieved from https://www.gov.uk/government/publications/womens-health-strategy-for-england.
18 Department of Health & Social Care (6 Mar. 2021). Government launches call for evidence to improve health and wellbeing of women in England. Retrieved from https://www.gov.uk/government/consultations/womens-health-strategy-call-for-evidence/womens-health-strategy-call-for-evidence.

CHAPTER 9: GAYNOR (PESSARIES AND 'VADGETS')

1 Downing, K. T. (2012). Uterine prolapse: From antiquity to today. *Obstetrics and Gynecology International*, 2012.
2 National Institute for Health and Care Excellence (9 Dec. 2021). Pelvic floor dysfunction: Prevention and non-surgical management. Recommendations. Retrieved from https://www.nice.org.uk/guidance/ng210/chapter/Recommendations.
3 Ibid.
4 Grand View Research (n.d.). Pelvic floor electric stimulator

market size, share & trends analysis report by application (urinary incontinence, neurodegenerative diseases, sexual dysfunction), by region, and segment forecasts, 2021– 2028. Retrieved from https://www.grandviewresearch.com/industry-analysis/pelvic-floor-electric-stimulator-market#:~:text=b.-,The%20global%20pelvic%20floor%20electric%20stimulator%20market%20size%20was%20valued,USD%20199.38%20million%20in%202021.&text=The%20global%20pelvic%20floor%20electric%20stimulator%20market%20is%20expected%20to,USD%20427.15%20million%20in%202028.

5 Partington, M. (19 Sep. 2021). Elvie's Tania Boler: Lessons in overcoming investors' resistance. *Financial Times*. Retrieved from https://www.ft.com/content/634ddd2f-ec11-4554-8979-5e631923d4e1.

CHAPTER 10: JAN (THE M WORD)

1 Harvard Health Publishing (13 Oct. 2021). Strength training builds more than muscles. Retrieved from https://www.health.harvard.edu/staying-healthy/strength-training-builds-more-than-muscles.

2 Liu, Y., Lee, D. C., Li, Y., Zhu, W., Zhang, R., Sui, X., et al (2019). Associations of resistance exercise with cardiovascular disease morbidity and mortality. *Medicine and Science in Sports and Exercise*, 51(3), 499.

3 NHS (9 Sep. 2019). Benefits and risks: Hormone replacement therapy. Retrieved from https://www.nhs.uk/conditions/hormone-replacement-therapy-hrt/risks/.

4 British Menopause Society (Sep. 2020). A woman's relationship with the menopause is complicated . . . [infographic]. Retrieved from https://thebms.org.uk/wp-content/uploads/2020/09/BMS-Infographic-A-womans-relationship-with-the-menopause-SEPT2020-B.pdf.

References

5 Short, H. (1 Apr. 2015). Let's talk menopause because we are failing 13 million women. *Guardian*. Retrieved from https://www.theguardian.com/healthcare-network/2015/apr/01/lets-talk-menopause-because-we-are-failing-13-million-women.

6 UK Parliament (28 Jul. 2022). New report: MPs call for new Menopause Ambassador to keep women in the workplace. Retrieved from https://committees.parliament.uk/committee/328/women-and-equalities-committee/news/172500/new-report-mps-call-for-new-menopause-ambassador-to-keep-women-in-the-workplace/.

7 National Institute for Health and Care Excellence (5 Dec. 2019). Menopause: Diagnosis and management. Retrieved from https://www.nice.org.uk/guidance/ng23.

8 Department for Education (2019). Relationships education, relationships and sex education (RSE) and health education. Retrieved from https://assets.publishing.service.gov.uk/government/uploads/system/uploads/attachment_data/file/1090195/Relationships_Education_RSE_and_Health_Education.pdf.

9 NHS Resolution (16 Jun. 2022). Vaginal mesh. Retrieved from https://resolution.nhs.uk/vaginal-mesh/.

10 The Independent Medicines and Medical Devices Safety Review (2020). *First Do No Harm*. Retrieved from https://www.immdsreview.org.uk/downloads/IMMDSReview_Web.pdf.

11 Ibid.

12 Hill, K. (1996). The demography of menopause. *Maturitas*, 23(2), 113–27.

13 GenM (n.d.). The GenM invisibility report. Retrieved from https://gen-m.com/wp-content/uploads/2021/09/106847-Gen-M-Invisibility-Report-082.pdf.

CHAPTER 11: POP CLUB! (FIND YOUR PEOPLE)

1 NHS (3 May 2019). Pudendal neuralgia. Retrieved from https://www.nhs.uk/conditions/pudendal-neuralgia/.
2 Marvel, R. P. (2018). Pudendal neuralgia: Making sense of a complex condition. *Current Sexual Health Reports*, 10(4), 237–45.
3 NHS (3 May 2019). Pudendal neuralgia. Retrieved from https://www.nhs.uk/conditions/pudendal-neuralgia/.

Acknowledgements

Massive thanks to my hugely talented agent, Kerry Glencorse, who convinced me that I could write this book and patiently guided me through every step of the process. Put simply, it wouldn't have happened without you. Thanks to my editor, Clare Drysdale, for your absolute belief and unwavering support, and to the rest of the team at Allen & Unwin – I will forever be grateful for your energy and encouragement. Thanks also to Julia Kellaway for your meticulous copy-editing and kind words.

To the brave and badass women who have trusted me with your stories and allowed me to share them, thank you. I will never underestimate what it took to speak out. You are pelvic floor warriors and are changing the world with your stigma-smashing honesty. Thanks also to the many experts who have given your time and wisdom so generously. And especially to the pelvic health physiotherapist, Emma Brockwell, who has not only cheered me on but also done a wonderful job of making sure that what I've written makes clinical sense!

To every medical and fitness professional who has helped to put me back together, piece by piece, over the years, thank you. You have been, and continue to be, a big part of this story. Thanks also to those family members and friends who persuaded me to keep writing when I got scared and wanted to stop. You know who you are.

My heartfelt thanks to Cat Pearson, for the beautiful illustrations, words of wisdom and friendship. You're an inspiration. I mean it. And to my husband, Paul, thanks for letting me share your life and your garden office; for the tech support and domestic wizardry; and for always, always believing.

Index

Index